PROGRESS IN CLINICAL AND BIOLOGICAL RESEARCH

RECENT TITLES

Please contact publisher for information about previous titles in this series.

DYNAMIC INTERACTIONS OF MYELIN PROTEINS

DYNAMIC INTERACTIONS OF MYELIN PROTEINS

Proceedings of a Symposium on Dynamic Interactions of Myelin Proteins, held in Chicago, Illinois, April 5–10, 1989

Editors

George A. Hashim
Surgical Research Labs
St. Luke's-Roosevelt Hospital Center
New York, New York

Mario Moscarello
Research Institute
The Hospital for Sick Children
Toronto, Ontario, Canada

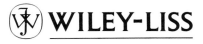

A JOHN WILEY & SONS, INC., PUBLICATION
NEW YORK • CHICHESTER • BRISBANE • TORONTO • SINGAPORE

Address all Inquiries to the Publisher
Wiley-Liss, Inc., 41 East 11th Street, New York, NY 10003

The publication of this volume was facilitated by the authors and editors who submitted the text in a form suitable for direct reproduction without subsequent editing or proofreading by the publisher.

Library of Congress Cataloging-in-Publication Data

Symposium on Dynamic Interaction of Myelin Proteins (1989 : Chicago, Ill.)
    Dynamic interactions of myelin proteins : proceedings of a Symposium on Dynamic Interaction of Myelin Proteins, held in Chicago, Illinois, April 5-10, 1989 / editors, George A. Hashim, Mario Moscarello.
        p.   cm. -- (Progress in clinical and biological research ; v. 336)
    Includes bibliographical references.
    ISBN 0-471-56729-9
    1. Myelin basic protein--Congresses.   2. Myelination--Congresses.
3. Myelin sheath--Congresses.   I. Hashim, George A.
II. Moscarello, Mario.   III. Title.   IV. Series.
    [DNLM: 1. Myelin Proteins--physiology--congresses.   2. Myelin Sheath--physiology--congresses.   W1 PR668E v. 336 / WL 102.5]
QP552.M88S96   1989
599.01'88--dc20
DNLM/DLC
for Library of Congress   89-70596
                                                              CIP

Contents

Contributors

Eugene D. Day, Department of Immunology, Duke University Medical Center, Durham, NC 27710 [109]

Jeffrey A. Hammer, Section on Myelin and Brain Development, NINDS, NIH, Bethesda, MD 20892 [49]

George Hashim, St. Luke's-Roosevelt Hospital and Columbia University, New York, NY 10021 [xi,93]

Leroy Hood, Division of Biology, California Institute of Technology, Pasadena, CA 91125 [81]

Gerhard Meissner, Department of Biochemistry and Nutrition, University of North Carolina School of Medicine, Chapel Hill, NC 27599 [1]

Pierre Morell, Department of Biochemistry and Nutrition, and Biological Sciences Research Center, University of North Carolina School of Medicine, Chapel Hill, NC 27599 [1]

Mario A. Moscarello, Research Institute, The Hospital for Sick Children, Toronto, Ontario, Canada M5G 1X8 [xi, 25]

Halina Offner, Department of Neurology, Oregon Health Sciences University, Portland, OR 97201 [93]

Brian Popko, Biological Sciences Research Center, University of North Carolina School of Medicine, Chapel Hill, NC 27599 [81]

Richard H. Quarles, Section on Myelin and Brain Development, NINDS, NIH, Bethesda, MD 20892 [49]

Carol Readhead, Division of Biology, California Institute of Technology, Pasadena, CA 91125 [81]

Michael D. Roberson, Department of Biochemistry and Nutrition, and Biological Sciences Research Center, University of North Carolina School of Medicine, Chapel Hill, NC 27599 [1]

H. David Shine, Center for Biotechnology, Baylor College of Medicine, Houston, TX 77030 [81]

Richard L. Sidman, Department of Neuropathology, Harvard Medical School, Boston, MA 02115 [81]

Arrel D. Toews, Department of Biochemistry and Nutrition, and Biological Sciences Research Center, University of North Carolina School of Medicine, Chapel Hill, NC 27599 [1]

The numbers in brackets are the opening page numbers of the contributors' articles.

Bruce D. Trapp, Department of
Neurology, The Johns Hopkins
University School of Medicine,
Baltimore, MD 21205 **[49]**

Arthur A. Vandenbark, Departments of
Neurology and Microbiology and
Immunology, Oregon Health Sciences
University, Portland, OR 97201 **[93]**

Preface

The stability and instability of myelin are evaluated by the dynamic interactions of the protein and lipid components of myelin membranes. How may these interactions lead to myelin stability and normal function, how may they lead to instability and abnormal function, and how may the metabolic processes, genetic imprints, or post-translational modifications lead to stability or instability of myelin membrane during development? Also, should instability be the outcome? What are the immunological responses that may be generated, and what kind of restrictions may be imposed on such responses? These are some of the issues we discuss in this book. We trust that the presentations will provoke further planning and experimentation designed to elucidate the principles put forth.

George A. Hashim, Ph.D.
Mario A. Moscarello, M.D.

Dynamic Interactions of Myelin Proteins, pages 1–23
© 1990 Alan R. Liss, Inc.

MYELIN: FROM ELECTRICAL INSULATOR TO ION CHANNELS

Pierre Morell, Michael D. Roberson, Gerhard
Meissner, and Arrel D. Toews

Department of Biochemistry and Nutrition, and
Biological Sciences Research Center (P.M.,
M.D.R., A.D.T.), University of North Carolina
School of Medicine, Chapel Hill, NC 27599-7250

INTRODUCTION

The realization that myelin serves as an electrical insulator was first articulated by Ranvier (1878). He postulated that myelin serves as an insulating sheath and "the transmission of sensory or motor impulses has some analogy with the transmission of electricity, and maybe it is convenient that each nerve tube is insulated so that this transmission is more effective" (quoted and discussed by Ritchie, 1984). Ranvier's speculation relating the function of myelin to insulation used in marine telegraph cables was far off the mark; propagation of impulses by a moving wave of depolarization across a membrane cannot be analyzed in terms of cable properties. He was, however, correct in that an assumption of negligible capacitance of myelin is basic to our present understanding of saltatory conduction, the discontinuous conduction of impulses along myelinated fibers.

A view of myelin as an insulator would not presuppose a need for active metabolism for this structure. The view of myelin as inert was in no way contradicted by detailed morphological and biophysical studies. A variety of bio-physical methods demonstrate that myelin is a multilamellar structure formed by successive spirals of plasma membrane which are tightly apposed against each other. Myelin is birefringent and thus has much ordered structure. It was difficult to conceive of how components of this membrane, arranged in this condensed layered structure, would have access to the cytoplasmic machinery presumably necessary for metabolism.

The data concerning the chemical composition of myelin also supports a view that this structure is specialized to form a relatively rigid bilayer. For a time it was even supposed that myelin was not a fluid mosaic in the same sense as other membranes, although it is now clear that most of the myelin is in a fluid mosaic state (Braun, 1984). Brain myelin, known to be the differentiated product of the plasma membrane of the oligodendroglial cell, has a chemical composition distinct from that of other plasma membrane derived fractions. It is notable for its high proportion of lipid (over 70% of its mass, compared to the 40 to 50% characteristic of most plasma membranes). Furthermore, these lipids include not only the typical plasma membrane content of cholesterol, 27%, but also large amounts of specialized lipids such as cerebroside, 24%, sulfatide, 7%, and ethanolamine plasmalogen, 15%; (Norton and Cammer, 1984). The latter three lipids are present at only low levels in other membranes.

The protein composition of myelin is also unusual. Almost half of myelin protein consists of a very hydrophobic protein, proteolipid protein, of apparent molecular weight 28,000, as well as a slightly smaller protein which is a splicing product of the same mRNA message. About a third consists of myelin basic proteins. The main form has an apparent molecular weight of about 18,000, but there are also several related proteins which are splicing products of the same mRNA message. The remainder consists of a number of higher molecular weight proteins, two of which, myelin associated glycoprotein and a cyclic nucleotide phospho-hydrolase, are well characterized in the myelin sheath and are presumed to play a special role in the development or function of myelin. This protein composition is in contrast with that defined for many other plasma membrane preparations of different cell types. Typically the protein composition of such membranes is very heterogeneous, with no single protein accounting for more than a few percent of the total. Thus it makes sense to view myelin as a specialized thick insulating sheath of lipid held in place by a relatively small amount of specialized protein.

METABOLIC TURNOVER

There is a large literature dealing with the use of isotopically labeled precursors of myelin components to study myelin metabolism (for review, see Benjamins and Smith, 1984). One aspect of this involves developmental studies and takes advantage of the fact that myelin deposition in rats and mice, the subjects of most metabolic studies, is a postnatal event. Myelin starts to be rapidly deposited at about 10 days of age; this is followed by a peak in the rate of accumulation at about 20 days, and then a gradual reduction in the rate of accumulation (Fig. 1). Thus, the rate of accumulation of myelin varies greatly during development. This is the basis for one approach to determine if a myelin component is metabolically stable. If a radioactive precursor is incorporated into a metabolically completely stable compound, then accumulation of radio-activity in that myelin component should be proportional to the rate of accumulation of that component. Assuming the composition of myelin does not change drastically over the time period in question, accumulation of radioactivity will also be proportional to the rate of accumulation of myelin. Such experiments can be done in vivo (following injection of the precursor) or in vitro (e.g., incubating brain slices from animals of various ages with radioactive precursor). Incorporation of radioactive precursor into metabolically stable myelin components is much more extensive during the period of rapid myelin deposition relative to the rate of incorporation at later ages. For example, incorporation of radioactive sugar into cerebroside (galactosylceramide) or of sulfur into sulfatide (galactosylceramide sulfate) closely follows the rate of myelin accumulation (Fig. 1).

Another type of experimental design gives a quanti-tative measure of metabolic half-life. In these experiments, animals are injected with a radioactive precursor and, following killing of animals at various times after injection, myelin is isolated and radioactivity remaining in particular myelin components determined. A plot of radioactivity remaining as a function of time allows direct calculation of apparent metabolic half-life. The earlier experiments of this type utilized time points of the order of weeks and months, leading to results which were compatible with an hypothesis of metabolic stability. A concept originally presented by Davison and co-workers (1964; 1965) and well substantiated by the available data at the time, was that turnover of myelin components was very slow - of the order of many months - and such turnover as did occur involved metabolism of myelin as a unit. Later experiments by Smith (1967; 1968) confirmed the relative metabolic

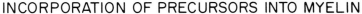
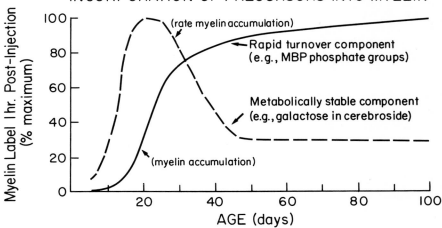

INCORPORATION OF PRECURSORS INTO MYELIN

(rate myelin accumulation)

Rapid turnover component
(e.g., MBP phosphate groups)

Metabolically stable component
(e.g., galactose in cerebroside)

(myelin accumulation)

Myelin Label 1hr. Post-Injection (% maximum)

AGE (days)

FIGURE 1.

stability of myelin but suggested that different structural
components did indeed turn over at different rates; the rates
determined ranged from weeks to months. Suggestions of even
more rapid turnover rates, of the order of days for some
myelin lipids, also appeared (Horrocks, 1969).

Another level of sophistication concerning metabolism
of myelin was arrived at by consideration of the metabolic
specificity of different radioactive precursors. For
example, the glycerol backbone of much of the myelin
phospholipid turns over relatively rapidly (of the order of a
few days), while the long chain acyl moieties are reutilized
and have much longer apparent turnover rates. Data on
turnover of myelin phosphatidylethanolamine in rats pulse-
labeled by intracranial injection of [2-^{3}H]glycerol at 17
days of age (Miller et al., 1977) is presented in Figure 2A.
The potential for confusing and contradictory conclusions (as
are amply present in the literature) is obvious - the
metabolic half life determined will be a function of which

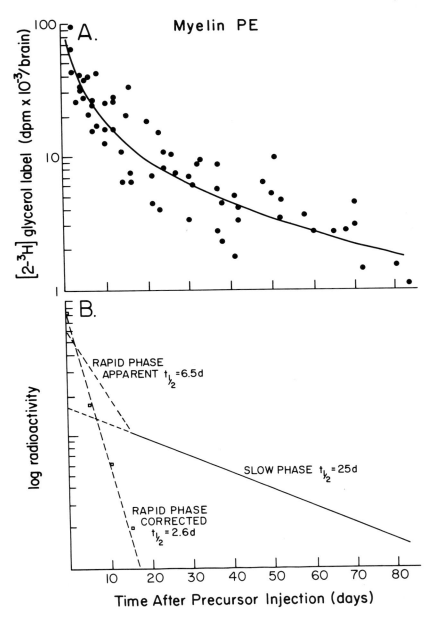

FIGURE 2.   Turnover of myelin phosphatidylethanolamine (PE).

time interval is examined. The data indicate that much of
the phosphatidylethanolamine synthesized during a period of
pulse-labeling (presumably the intracranially injected
[2-^{3}H]glycerol is only available for a time period of the
order of minutes before it is utilized, degraded, or loses
the tritium label from the C-2 position by the action of
glycerolphosphate dehydrogenase) is metabolized rapidly. In
Figure 2B, the decay of label in phosphatidylethanolamine is
arbitrarily resolved into two phases. Although many phases
could be contributing to the shape of the curve, it seems
evident that a significant portion of the total myelin lipid
does turn over with a half life of the order of days or
faster. It is possible to calculate the amount of PE in the
"slow" and "fast" pools through a quantitative analysis
described by Horrocks et al. (1976). By this calculation,
38% of the phosphatidylethanolamine is in the fast pool and
62% is in the slow pool.

The nature of the slowly and the more rapidly turning
over pools with respect to morphological parameters is not
clear - there is no strong data to identify, for example, the
outer or inner layers of the sheath as containing lipid
preferentially in one or the other pool. A question arising
is how some myelin glycerolipids may be metabolically stable
while others are rapidly metabolized. If the entire membrane
is a rapidly equilibrating fluid mosaic, then all myelin
lipids of the same molecular composition should be
equivalent. Perhaps subtle differences in fatty acyl
composition determine metabolic turnover of individual lipid
species (the experimental protocols generally used in such
turnover studies do not resolve intact molecular species of
individual lipid classes). Another possibility is that all
parts of the same myelin membrane are not in equilibrium.
Braun (1984) comments that "the high relative proportion of
cholesterol in the external half of the bilayer, possibly
approaching 'saturating' levels, suggests that nonhomogeneous
distribution of 'patches' cannot be ruled out". The apparent
turnover rate also varies with the age of the animals when
injected with radioactive precursor; as the rate of
deposition of myelin decreases during later development,
total incorporation of label decreases and an ever larger
proportion of incorporated label is in the rapidly turning
over metabolic compartment (Miller and Morell, 1978).

Although the availability of data concerning turnover
of myelin components is greater for lipids than for proteins,

the situation for myelin proteins seems to be similar (Lajtha et al., 1977; see Benjamins and Smith, 1984 for review). Different myelin proteins turn over at different rates; myelin proteolipid and basic proteins are more stable than many of the higher molecular weight proteins. The data discussed above, although indicating metabolic activity for myelin, do not challenge an assumption that myelin must play a relatively passive role in its function of facilitating propagation of impulses along the axon.

A question now under investigation is the possible presence of an extremely rapidly turning over metabolic compartment within myelin. It has been demonstrated (DesJardins and Morell, 1983) that the phosphate groups which posttranslationally modify the myelin basic proteins turn over very rapidly. The experiments demonstrating this rapid turnover involved intracranial injection of [^{33}P]phosphate. It was shown that much of the phosphate which covalently modifies the basic proteins of compact myelin was rapidly replaced by radioactive phosphate. The turnover is of the order of minutes or faster (the in vivo methodology utilized depended on the conversion of injected radioactive phosphate to radioactive ATP, and thus the temporal resolution was limited). In addition, the injected [^{33}P]phosphate rapidly exchanged with phosphate groups on the basic proteins in pre-existing mature myelin (adult brain) to the same extent as in younger animals, where the processes of myelin synthesis and compaction are occurring at high levels. Figure 3 compares incorporation of [^{33}P]phosphate and [^{3}H]glycine into myelin basic proteins one hour after injection in 18, 30, and 60 day old rats. The incorporation of glycine reflects the rate of synthesis of the peptide backbone of the basic proteins and as expected, incorporation (expressed per mg myelin protein) was highest at 18 days of age and declined markedly with increasing age. In marked contrast, incorporation of [^{33}P]phosphate into the basic proteins, expressed in the same manner, was the same at all three ages. Thus, incorporation of phosphate was not proportional to the rate of myelin synthesis, but was rather proportional to the total amount of myelin present (see Fig. 1). This very rapid turnover implies that the compacted myelin is not a static structure but that, somehow, enzyme activity and substrates involved in the covalent modification of proteins are available. One interpretation is that the compaction of the cytoplasmic faces of the myelin sheath (evident by electron microscopic and other biophysical techniques) can be overcome by

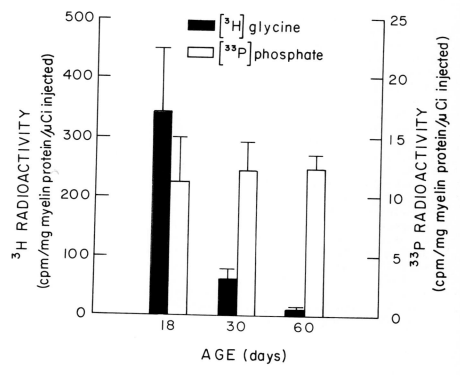

FIGURE 3. Sixty minutes after intracranial injection of
[2-³H]glycerol and [³³P]orthophosphate, myelin was isolated,
proteins separated by gel electrophoresis, and radioactivity
in basic proteins determined (DesJardins and Morell, 1983).

metabolic processes making for the momentary appearance of
cytoplasmic pockets within compact myelin. Existence of such
a metabolic compartment also suggests the possibility that
myelin does not play strictly a passive role with respect to
movement of information along the axon.

PHOSPHOINOSITIDE METABOLISM

One aspect of myelin metabolism, well documented some
two decades ago (Sheltawy and Dawson, 1969), is the rapid
incorporation of [³²P]phosphate into the polyphosphoinositides
of myelin. This observation has been verified in a tissue

slice system (Deshmukh et al, 1978). A quantitative study of the metabolism of myelin polyphosphoinositides has been carried out using rat brain slices (Kahn and Morell, 1988). After a one hour incubation in the presence of radioactive phosphate, over 30% of the total radioactivity in phosphatidic acid (PA), 13% of the total radioactivity in phosphatidylinositol bisphosphate (PIP_2), and 7% of that in phosphatidylinositol phosphate (PIP), was present in myelin. On a per mg protein basis, PA labeling in myelin is 2.5-fold greater than in whole brain slices, and it is clear that at least some of the polyphosphoinositides, which are enriched in myelin, are rapidly labeled. Since incorporation of radioactive glycerol into myelin PA and polyphosphoinositides is negligible (and much lower than incorporation into the corresponding non-myelin lipids), it was concluded that incorporation of ^{32}P-label into PA and PI involved phospholipase C action. Further analysis of the data suggested that much of the label in polyphosphoinositides was there as a result of turnover of the monoesterified phosphate groups on the inositol moiety. This somewhat indirect evidence for phospholipase C activity is of interest in the context that a product of this reaction, diglyceride, is known to stimulate protein kinase C and, in turn, this kinase (known to be present in myelin, Miyamoto, 1975) may be involved in control of ion channel activity.

Not only is there vigorous metabolism of the phosphoinositides; it appears that this aspect of metabolic turnover is cholinergically stimulated (Kahn and Morell, 1988; Larocca et al., 1987a). It has been demonstrated that the presence of acetylcholine in the incubation medium for brain slices accelerates incorporation of radioactive phosphate into the myelin phosphoinositides (Kahn and Morell, 1988). Cholinergically stimulated turnover implies the presence of receptors in myelin and this has recently been demonstrated (Larocca et al., 1987b). Another component expected to be associated with ligand-stimulated phosphoinositide metabolism is a set of G proteins. Indeed, recent reports suggest the presence of GTP-binding proteins in isolated myelin (Bernier et al., 1989). The available evidence is, therefore, supportive of a system allowing for cholinergic stimulation of phosphoinositide metabolism in myelin.

ION CHANNELS IN MYELIN

As noted in the introduction, the common view regarding the function of myelin is that it serves primarily as an interrupted insulator. The evidence for a rapid metabolic compartment within myelin, particularly that suggesting cholinergically-stimulated phosphoinositide metabolism, is difficult to integrate into this conventional view of the myelin sheath. In fact, stimulated phosphoinositide metabolism is often correlated with the presence of ion channels and a system for control of their activity. In addition, several other lines of evidence also suggest the possibility of ion channels in myelin. These include the presence in myelin of enzymes which regulate ion transport (carbonic anhydrase, Cammer, 1979; Na^+,K^+-ATPase, Reiss et al., 1981; protein kinases, Miyamoto, 1975) and the reported ionophoric properties of certain myelin proteins (Lin and Lees, 1982; Cheifetz et al., 1985; Fischer et al., 1989).

We have initiated a research program to determine whether myelin does indeed contain ion channels. The basic experimental approach we utilize to test this hypothesis is to create myelin vesicles and to test for ion flux across the vesicle membrane. Our initial expectation was that we would be able to make single bilayer vesicles, since there are two reports of such preparations in the literature. In our hands, however, the procedure reported by Steck et al. (1978) does not provide a preparation of single bilayer vesicles – our failure to replicate this procedure is documented in a previous publication (Sedzik et al., 1984). We also attempted to replicate the production of unilamellar vesicles as outlined in a more recent publication by Lin et al. (1986). Although in our hands this procedure did significantly reduce the size and number of lamellae of the myelin particles, it also did not produce a significant yield of unilamellar vesicles as monitored by electron microscopy. We continue to explore protocols for production of unilamellar vesicles from myelin.

Our initial ion channel experiments have utilized a preparation procedure (Fig. 4) which, by visual inspection of electron micrographs (Fig. 5), gives a relatively good yield of "vesicles." However, when these preparations were examined at very high magnification, it was apparent that much of the preparation consisted of structures with one to three major dense lines (presumably two to six membrane

DAY 1

Homogenize brain in 0.32 M sucrose

Isolate myelin (Norton and Poduslo, 1973)
sucrose gradient;
osmotic shock;
sucrose gradient

Incubate purified myelin overnight in
1 mM phosphate buffer, 1 mM EGTA, pH 8.0

DAY 2

Equilibrate at 2000 psi N_2 for
30 min in cell disruption bomb

Release pressure rapidly
to disrupt lamellae and
form vesicles

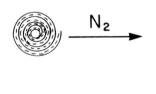 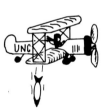 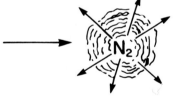

Concentrate by centrifugation; pass through 25 gauge needle;
Equilibrate for 3 hrs with equal volume of 0.5 M sucrose

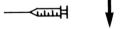

Centrifuge at 12,000 x g for 10 min;
Save supernatant in tube labeled "Myelin Vesicles"

FIGURE 4. Preparation of myelin "vesicles".

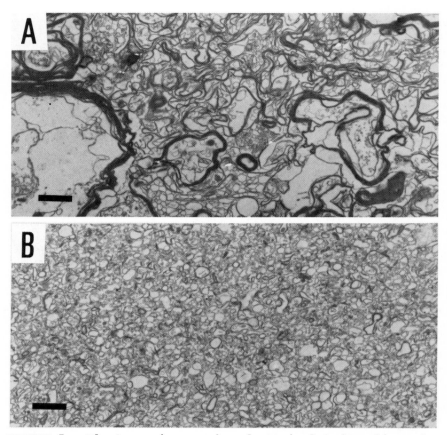

FIGURE 5. Electron micrographs of (A) isolated myelin and (B) "myelin vesicle" fraction prepared as described in Figure 4. Bar = 1 μm.

bilayers). The protocol involved preparation of myelin from the brains of sixty day old Long-Evans rats, utilizing the procedure of Norton and Poduslo (1973). The isolated myelin was then resuspended in 1mM phosphate buffer adjusted to pH 8.0 and containing 1 mM EGTA. The particulate myelin preparation was kept in suspension by gentle stirring for 16 h at 4°C. The myelin suspension was then equilibrated with nitrogen at 2000 psi in a cell disruption bomb and released rapidly to atmospheric pressure to disrupt lamellae and form vesicles (Lin et al., 1986). The myelin was again collected

by centrifugation at 85,000g for 30 min. and then resuspended
by being taken up into a hypodermic syringe and expelled
repeatedly through a 25 gauge needle. This preparation was
then equilibrated for three hours with sucrose at a final
concentration of 0.25 M. The material remaining in a
supernatant after centrifugation at 12,000g for ten minutes
was utilized as the "myelin vesicle" preparation. We
utilized three different approaches to investigate the ion
transport properties of this vesiculated myelin preparation.

Vesicle-Lipid Bilayer Fusion Studies

        In this experimental approach (Rosseau et al., 1988;
for review, see White, 1986), a planar lipid bilayer formed
from a mixture of phosphatidlyethanolamine, phosphatidylserine, and phosphatidylcholine (5:3:2 molar ratio),
separates two chambers containing isoosmolar K^+ (Fig. 6A).
Vesicles can be added to one of the chambers and eventually
such a vesicle, and any channels which it contains, may
spontaneously fuse with the planar lipid bilayer (Fig. 6B).
If a constant transmembrane potential is maintained between
the two chambers, the fusion of a channel-containing vesicle
will allow for flow of ions which can be monitored as abrupt
changes in transmembrane conductance corresponding to the
passage of single ions. Conductance of K^+ was almost always
evident after addition of the myelin vesicle preparation
(Fig. 6C). These results were encouraging, since they did
indeed support a conclusion that our preparation included
membranes containing K^+ channels. It is not, however,
possible to conclude that the channels are present in myelin
membranes. As noted, most of the membrane present has two or
more major dense lines and is therefore not unilamellar.
Questions arise as to what contaminating membrane fragments
might be present and what the efficiency of their fusion with
the planar lipid bilayer, relative to that of myelin, might
be. Although it has been repeatedly demonstrated that myelin
prepared by the procedure of Norton and Poduslo (1973) is 95%
or more pure, it is not possible to eliminate the possibility
of a few percent contamination from other brain membranes.
It may be that the small amount of truly unilamellar vesicles
preferentially represents non-myelin material, and that these
contaminating vesicles fuse preferentially with the planar
lipid bilayer. The presence of channels in myelin could also
be unambiguously established, even in the presence of
contaminating membranes, if channels present in the myelin

A.

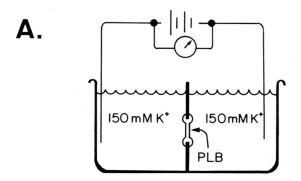

Vesicles are added to one of two chambers containing isoosmolar K+ and separated by a planar lipid bilayer (**PLB**), across which a constant transmembrane potential can be established.

B.

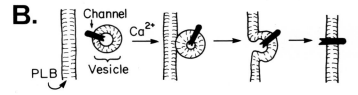

A channel is incorporated into the planar lipid bilayer when a channel—containing vesicle fuses with the bilayer.

C.

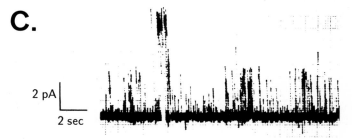

A recording of channel activity after fusion of a vesicle from the "myelin vesicle preparation" with the PLB. Channel activity (opening and closing) is evident as abrupt, minute changes in transmembrane conductance when current, in the form of K+ ions, passes through the open channel.

FIGURE 6. Vesicle-Lipid Bilayer Fusion Studies

preparation had unique properties (e.g., voltage gating different from that of other K^+ channels). Preliminary studies indicated that K^+ channels found in the myelin preparation were similar to those in many other brain membrane fractions, and thus this approach to demonstration of ion channels in myelin has been temporarily abandoned.

Isotope Efflux Studies

In this experimental paradigm (for review, see Meissner, 1988), vesicles are passively loaded with "permeant" and "impermeant" labeled compounds. The assumption is that, over a period of 12 to 16 hours, even a large hydrophilic molecule such as a sugar will diffuse across the vesicle membrane and equilibrate with the interior aqueous space. Small charged ions such as K^+ (or in this case $^{86}Rb^+$, which mimics K^+ with respect to transfer through specific ion channels) will also equilibrate with the internal aqueous space of vesicles. The two classes of molecules will, however, differ with respect to the rate at which they leave the vesicles after dilution with unlabeled incubation medium. If ion channels are present, the ions can exit the vesicle extremely rapidly with a time course of the order of a second or two. In contrast, the "impermeant" sugar could only equilibrate by the same diffusion process by which it entered the vesicle, with a time frame of minutes to hours. Thus, the apparent vesicle volume determined with respect to the sugar will be greater than that determined for the ion by that fraction of total vesicle volume which contains channels allowing for the very rapid efflux of the ion. Figure 7 outlines the experimental protocol and illustrates data of typical experiments performed to assay for the presence of Rb^+ channel activity, which presumably represents K^+ channels. The interpretation of this particular experiment depends on the assumption that most of the vesicles are passively loaded with mannitol and then retain it during dilution of the vesicles and for at least a few minutes after dilution. The vesicle space for $^{86}Rb^+$, as extrapolated to zero time without consideration of the presumed rapid efflux of ion before the first measurement, is less than half that of the mannitol space and indicates that this fraction of the vesicle volume rapidly equilibrates with the extravesicular space by one or more ion "channels." A series of such experiments have also been carried out using radioactive potassium and sodium ions; all the data are

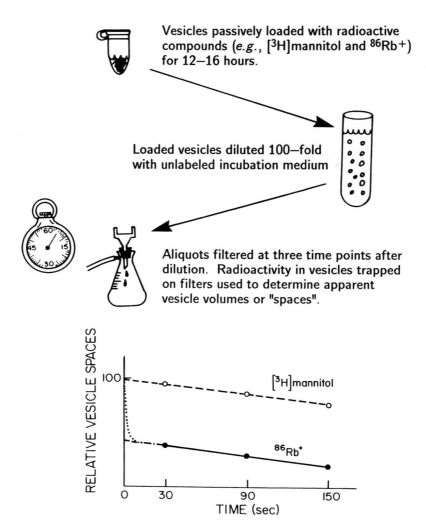

Vesicles passively loaded with radioactive compounds (*e.g.*, [³H]mannitol and ⁸⁶Rb⁺) for 12–16 hours.

Loaded vesicles diluted 100–fold with unlabeled incubation medium

Aliquots filtered at three time points after dilution. Radioactivity in vesicles trapped on filters used to determine apparent vesicle volumes or "spaces".

Assuming complete equilibration for both compounds with the interior of all vesicles, vesicle spaces at zero time are, in principle, identical. Differences in spaces determined by linear extrapolation to zero time are because much of the ⁸⁶Rb⁺ leaves vesicles "instantly" through "channels" while [³H]mannitol remains trapped.

FIGURE 7. Isotope Efflux Studies

supportive of the conclusion that about half of the total
mannitol-impermeable vesicle space is readily permeable to K^+
and Na^+ ions.

These studies, although still in a relatively preliminary stage, are encouraging. It should be noted that, in
contrast to the vesicle-lipid bilayer fusion studies
described in the previous section, assay of vesicle space is
a bulk phenomenon unlikely to be seriously perturbed by a
small fraction of contaminating membranes. A potential
defect in this approach is that, lacking demonstration of
specificity with respect to ion channels (i.e., an ion which
is retained within the vesicles and does not leave rapidly)
the possibility exists that the membranes are slightly
damaged in such a way that larger molecules are retained but
small molecules are nonspecifically allowed to leak out
rapidly.

Light-Scattering Studies

This methodology (Fig. 8; for review, see Meissner,
1988) involves equilibration of vesicles in a low osmolarity
buffer during which the vesicles presumably attain a
spherical shape. The vesicles are then subjected to a
hyperosmotic environment by addition of a concentrated
solution of solute. If the vesicles are impermeable to the
solute, they rapidly lose water due to the higher osmotic
pressure of the solute. The consequent change in size and
shape of the vesicles leads to an increase in light-
scattering. The increased light-scattering seen upon
addition of the hyperosmotic solute is attenuated to the
extent that the vesicles are permeable to the added solute;
this is because the solute enters so rapidly that there is
less loss of water and less accompanying changes in vesicle
size and shape.

Preliminary results of light-scattering experiments
utilizing a "myelin vesicle" preparation are shown in Figure
9. In these experiments, effects of $KHCO_3$ were compared with
those of mannitol, which was used as the "impermeable"
solute. The response to added $KHCO_3$ was not markedly less
than that seen upon addition of the impermeable mannitol.
Furthermore, this response to $KHCO_3$ was not altered by the
presence of valinomycin, a K^+-ionophore which should allow
unrestricted entry of K^+ ions into the vesicles. These

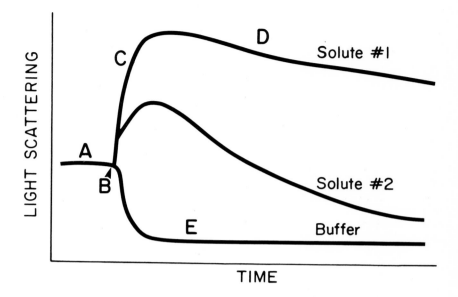

Equilibrate vesicles in low osmolarity buffer. Transfer to cuvette in fluorometer and achieve steady baseline (**A**)

Addition of hyperosmotic solution (**B**) causes vesicle shrinkage.

As vesicles impermeable to solute lose water and shrink, light scattering increases (**C**).

Shrunken vesicles slowly regain original shape and size as solutes and water enter; light scattering decreases (**D**).

Dilution of vesicles upon addition of hyperosmotic solution simultaneously reduces light scattering response. Equivalent dilution with isoosmotic buffer creates new lower control baseline (**E**).

Submaximal response (amplitudes) and faster recovery (slopes) indicate differences in permeability of vesicles to various solutes. In the example above, solute #2 is more permeable than solute #1.

FIGURE 8. Light Scattering Studies

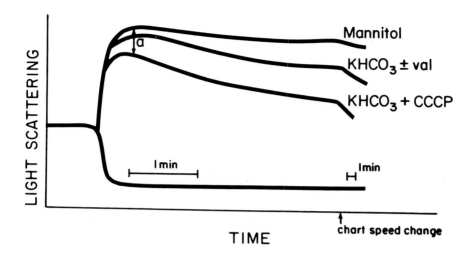

FIGURE 9. Light scattering by a myelin "vesicle" preparation

findings suggest that poor permeability to the HCO_3^- counter-ion may be the rate-limiting factor. The entry of HCO_3^- into the vesicles is in some way aided by addition of carbonyl cyanide m-chlorophenyl-hydrazone (CCCP), a proton ionophore which facilitates the recovery of vesicles hyperosmotically collapsed with $KHCO_3$. How might a proton ionophore aid HCO_3^- entry? It is possible that the bicarbonate counter-ion diffuses into the vesicles as free CO_2 (following combination with a proton to form carbonic acid, which dissociates into free CO_2 and water). The reverse reaction, combination of CO_2 and H_2O to yield carbonic acid, inside the vesicles would yield, upon dissociation, HCO_3^- and a proton. The presence of a proton ionophore could aid HCO_3^- formation and K^+ inward movement by permitting H^+ efflux. We note that the myelin proteolipid protein (PLP) may play a similar role under physiological conditions, since it is known to have proton transport properties (Lin and Lees, 1982). It is not known why, under our conditions of efflux assay, the proteolipid protein in the vesicles is not acting as a good proton ionophore (apparently it is not active, since the addition of the known proton ionophore, CCCP, alters the light scattering rather significantly).

The scheme proposed above suggests a functional role for carbonic anhydrase in myelin. This enzyme, which catalyzes conversion of CO_2 and H_2O to carbonic acid, is prominent in myelin (Cammer, 1979). Also of potential interest is the recent report that the K^+-channel forming plasma membrane proteolipid protein is present in myelin (Fischer et al., 1989).

CONCLUSIONS

Much of the myelin membrane is metabolically stable; the biochemical or structural basis for this is not known. Even within the compacted myelin sheath, however, there is significant turnover of many of the membrane components. In addition, there is a very rapid turnover of some moieties of myelin components - the phosphate groups of inositol phospholipids and of myelin basic proteins. These demonstrations of dynamic metabolism, some of which may be related to ligand-stimulated second messenger systems, suggest the possibility that myelin may participate actively in the process of conduction of information along the axon. We suggest that this role may involve the compartmentalization of potassium. The possible involvement of myelin in compartmentalization of K^+ is supported by the results of several biophysical techniques which suggest the presence of K^+ "channels" in isolated myelin "vesicles."

ACKNOWLEDGEMENTS

These studies were supported in part by USPHS grants NS-11615 and HD-03110. We thank Nelson D. Goines for assistance with the electron microscopy and photography.

REFERENCES

Adams CWM, Davison AN (1965). The myelin sheath. In Adams CWM (ed): "Neurohistochemistry," Amsterdam: Elsevier, pp 332-400.
Benjamins JA, Smith ME (1984). Metabolism of myelin. In Morell P (ed): "Myelin", New York: Plenum Press, pp 225-258.
Bernier L, Hovrath E, Braun P (1989). GTP binding proteins in CNS myelin. Trans Amer Soc Neurochem 20:254.

Braun PE (1984). Molecular organization of myelin. In
    Morell P (ed): "Myelin", New York: Plenum Press, pp 97–
    116.
Cammer W (1979). Carbonic anhydrase activity in myelin from
    sciatic nerves of adult and young rats: quantitation and
    inhibitor sensitivity. J Neurochem 32:651–654.
Cheifetz S, Boggs JM, Moscarello MA (1985). Increase in
    vesicle permeability mediated by myelin basic protein.
    Bioc 24:5170–5175.
Davison AN (1964). Myelin metabolism. In (Dawson RMC, Rhodes
    DN (eds): "Metabolism and Physiological Significance of
    Lipids," London: Wiley, pp 527–540.
Deshmukh DS, Bear WD, Brockerhoff H (1978). Polyphospho-
    inositide biosynthesis in three subfractions of rat brain
    myelin. J Neurochem 30:1191–1193.
DesJardins KC, Morell P (1983). The phosphate groups
    modifying myelin basic proteins are metabolically labile;
    the methyl groups are stable. J Cell Biol 97:438–446.
Fischer I, Cochary E, Bizzozero O, Sapirstein V (1989). The
    plasma membrane proteolipid is enriched in myelin. Trans
    Amer Soc Neurochem 20:257.
Horrocks LA (1969). Metabolism of the ethanolamine phospho-
    glycerides of mouse brain myelin and microsomes. J
    Neurochem 16:13–18.
Horrocks LA, Toews AD, Thompson DK, Chin JY (1976).
    Synthesis and turnover of brain phosphoglycerides –
    results, methods of calculation and interpretation. In
    Porcellati G, Amaducci L, Galli C (eds): "Function and
    Metabolism of Phospholipids in the Central and Peripheral
    Nervous Systems," New York: Plenum Press, pp 37–54.
Kahn DW, Morell P (1988). Phosphatidic acid and phospho-
    inositide turnover in myelin and its stimulation by
    acetylcholine. J Neurochem 50:1542–1550.
Lajtha A, Toth J, Fujimoto K, Agrawal HC (1977). Turnover of
    myelin proteins in mouse brain in vivo. Biochem J 164:323–
    329.
Larocca JN, Cervone A, Ledeen R (1987a). Stimulation of
    phosphoinositide hydrolysis in myelin by muscarinic
    agonist and potassium. Brain Res 436:357–362.
Larocca JN, Ledeen R, Dvorkin B, Makman MH (1987b).
    Muscarinic receptor binding and muscarinic receptor-
    mediated inhibition of adenylate cyclase in rat brain
    myelin. J Neurosci 7:3869–3876.
Lin L-FH, Bartlett C, Lees MB (1986). Preparation and
    characterization of unilamellar myelin vesicles. J Biol
    Chem 261:16241–16246.

Lin L-FH, Lees MB (1982). Interactions of dicyclohexyl-carbodiimide with myelin proteolipid. Proc Natl Acad Sci USA 79:941-945.

Meissner G (1988). Ionic permeability of isolated muscle sarcoplasmic reticulum and liver endoplasmic reticulum vesicles. In Fleischer S and Fleischer B (eds): "Methods in Enzymology, Volume 157, Biomembranes, Part Q, ATP-Driven Pumps and Related Transport: Calcium, Proton, and Potassium Pumps," New York: Academic Press, pp 417-437.

Miller SL, Benjamins JA, Morell P (1977). Metabolism of glycerophospholipids of myelin and microsomes in rat brain: Reutilization of precursors. J Biol Chem 252:4025-4037.

Miller SL, Morell P (1978). Turnover of phosphatidylcholine in microsomes and myelin in brains of young and adult rats. J Neurochem 31:771-777.

Miyamoto E (1975). Protein kinases in myelin of rat brain: solubilization and characterization. J Neurochem 24:503-512.

Norton WT, Cammer W (1984). Isolation and characterization of myelin. In Morell P (ed): "Myelin", New York: Plenum Press, pp 147-195.

Norton WT, Poduslo SE (1973). Myelination in rat brain: method of myelin isolation. J Neurochem 21:749-757.

Ranvier ML (1878). Leçons sur l'Histologie du Système Nerveux. Librairie F. Savy, Paris.

Reiss DS, Lees MB, Sapirstein VS (1981). Is Na + K ATPase a myelin-associated enzyme? J Neurochem 36:1418-1426.

Ritchie JM (1984). Physiological basis of conduction in myelinated nerve fibers. In Morell P (ed): "Myelin", New York: Plenum Press, pp 117-145.

Rosseau E, Roberson M, Meissner G (1988). Properties of single chloride selective channel from sarcoplasmic reticulum. Eur Biophys J 16:143-151.

Sedzik J, Toews AD, Blaurock AE, Morell P (1984). Resistance to disruption of multilamellar fragments of central nervous system myelin. J Neurochem 43:1415-1420.

Sheltawy A, Dawson RMC (1969). The metabolism of polyphosphoinositides in hen brain and sciatic nerve. Biochem J 111:157-165.

Smith ME (1967). The metabolism of myelin lipids. Adv Lipid Res 5:241-278.

Smith ME (1968). The turnover of myelin in the adult rat. Biochim Biophys Acta 164:285-293.

Steck AJ, Siegrist P, Zahler P, Herschkowitz NN, Schaefer R (1978). Preparation of membrane vesicles from isolated myelin. Studies on functional and structural properties. Biochim Biophys Acta 509:397–409.
White SH (1986). The physical nature of planar bilayer membranes. In Miller C (ed): "Ion Channel Reconstitution," pp 3–35.

Dynamic Interactions of Myelin Proteins, pages 25–48
© 1990 Alan R. Liss, Inc.

MYELIN BASIC PROTEIN : A DYNAMICALLY CHANGING
STRUCTURE

M. A. Moscarello

Research Institute
The Hospital for Sick Children Toronto, Canada
M5G 1X8

INTRODUCTION

The myelin sheath is the membranous structure which surrounds
the axons. It is composed of proteins and lipids in a ratio of roughly 1 to
4. The integrity of the myelin sheath depends upon non covalent
interactions between the proteins and lipids, primarily electrostatic and
hydrophobic types. Electrostatic interactions depend on the nature,
number and distribution of the charged groups along the protein
structure. The primary structure of the protein, i.e. the linear sequence of
amino acids is fixed by the genetic code so that the nature, number and
distribution of charge groups of the amino acids is fixed. On the other
hand, post translational modifications represent the final covalent
modification of proteins which impart to the protein its mature function
and provide a mechanism for change as a result of various metabolic
reactions. When the changes involve a charged group such as phosphate
the net charge on the protein changes with or without subsequent changes
in the folded structure. Changes in the latter may enhance not only
electrostatic interactions, but also hydrophobic interactions in the
membrane environment. The experiments presented below with myelin
basic protein (MBP) will demonstrate how post translational
modifications affect protein charge, structure and interactions in the
myelin membrane in an effort to dispel the static view of myelin,
prevalent until recently.

Studies of primary structure and protein lipid interactions have
resulted in the concept that MBP, because of its large positive charge
imparted to the molecule by 12 lysyl and 19 arginyl residues, functions
primarily to appose adjacent bilayers to form a compact myelin sheath
(BOGGS et al, 1982; RUMSBY, 1987). This concept is in keeping
with a model of the myelin sheath, functioning primarily as an insulator.

However, in recent years a more dynamic view of myelin has been gaining prominence without usurping its traditional role as an insulator. In support of this new concept, the discovery of a number of enzymes in or associated with myelin suggest a metabolically active membrane (NORTON and CAMMER, 1984). The presence of enzymes suggests the presence of substrates as well. Although many of the enzymes are lipid associated, a number of enzymes such as protein kinases, ribosyltransferases, methylases, etc. use MBP as a substrate. The product of these various reactions is a highly modified MBP molecule. Some of these post translational modifications give rise to charge microheterogeneity (e.g. phosphorylation) while others (e.g. methylation) do not. Profound changes have been documented, both in the folded structure of the protein, in its ability to interact with lipids, in its ability to induce EAE in susceptible animals and in development as a result of these various changes. Since MBP is the only myelin protein for which these various activities have been correlated, it will be considered in some detail.

Microheterogeneity of MBP was first demonstrated by MARTENSON, DEIBLER and KIES in 1969. Thus MBP which migrated as a single band on SDS-PAGE was resolved into multiple bands on urea gels at pH 10.6, some of which were purified by CM-52 chromatography also in urea at pH 10.6 (DEIBLER and MARTENSON, 1973). The source of this charge microheterogeneity was ascribed to deamidation, phosphorylation and the loss of a C-terminal arginine. The various protein fractions were termed components. Component 1 (C-1) was the most cationic and eluted last from the column. It was also considered the most unmodified. Component 2 (C-2) was thought to arise by deamidation of an amide and therefore contained one positive charge less than C-1. Component 3 (C-3) was shown to contain some phosphate although the amount was well below 1 mole/mole of protein which would be the amount required to impart two negative charges to the molecule e.g. MIYAMOTO and KAKIUCHI, 1974 reported 0.2 mol PO_4/mole MBP. Therefore the microheterogeneity of C-3 must be attributed to a combination of factors including phosphorylation, deamidation etc. In total as many as 8-10 charge isomers have been detected but most have not been characterized. The functional significance of this rather extensive charge microheterogeneity is only beginning to be understood. Some promising paths to follow will be described below.

Our interest in this problem was stimulated by two observations, one from our laboratory (CHEIFETZ and MOSCARELLO, 1985; CHEIFETZ*et al,* 1985) and one reported by Murray and Steck, 1984. In the latter experiments, phosphorylation of MBP was reported to accompany the conduction of an impulse along the optic nerve in vitro.

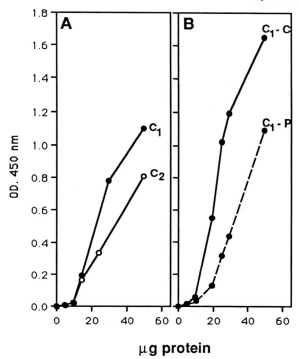

Fig 1   Vesicle Aggregation by C-1, C-2 from MBP and
         Phosphorylated C-1. Vesicles, composed of
         phosphatidylcholine and phosphatidylserine (92.2% PC and
         7.8% PS) were incubated with varying amounts of protein at
         R.T. for 15 min. The turbidity of 450 nm was measured. C_1 -
         component 1; C_2 - component 2; C_1 - C -represents C-1 after
         incubation in phosphorylating medium without ATP; C1-P
         phosphorylated
         C-1.

To my knowledge this interesting observation has not been followed up.
The reports from our laboratory showed that phosphorylation of C-1
markedly decreased its ability to interact with lipids in a vesicle
aggregation assay (Fig 1) and that phosphorylation of MBP disrupted the
bilayer sufficiently to alter the permeability of lipid vesicles to entrapped
spin label. From these studies we concluded that phosphorylation
affected both structural and functional properties of lipid vesicles.

These observations prompted us to begin a systematic study of microheterogeneity of MBP both that found naturally and induced in vitro by specific enzymes. In this way the effects of specific post translational modifications of MBP on the folded structure of MBP and the effects of some of these modifications on protein-lipid interactions, could be studied.

Phosphorylation

Several of the components of human MBP (or charge isomers, a more descriptive term) were phosphorylated by a protein Kinase C from brain. The extent of phosphorylation of C-1→ C-4 is shown in Table 1, which varied from 2.8±0.6 - 5.2±0.8 moles PO_4/mole MBP for the different components. Interestingly, phosphorylation of C-1 was the lowest at 2.8 moles PO_4/mole protein, even though it is considered to be the most unmodified of the components. Components 3 and 4 incorporated 3.2 and 5.2 moles PO_4/mole protein although both are partially phosphorylated as isolated. The effect of phosphorylation on the mobility of the protein in the alkaline-urea gel system is shown in Fig 2. When C-1 was phosphorylated, the mobility decreased to that expected of C-3. the mobilities of all other components changed in a corresponding fashion.

The effect of phosphorylation on the folded structure of the protein was studied next (RAMWANI et al, 1989). From the CD spectra the relative proportions of α−helix, β-structure, random structure and turns were obtained. The isolated, non phosphorylated components 1, 2 and 3 showed low proportions of -structure, from 0.13 - 0.19 while component 4 was higher at 0.24 (Table 2). The calculations for C-1 and

TABLE 1. Phosphorylation of human MBP charge isomers with human brain soluble Protein kinase C*

Charge Isomer	molPO4/ mol protein
C-1	2.8 ± 0.6[≠]
C-2	3.7 ± 0.5
C-3	3.2 ± 0.5
C-4	5.2 ± 0.8

*For phosphorylation, 50 μg of each component were incubated at 30° in a final volume of 200 μl containing 20 mM Tris buffer pH 7.5, 10 mM $MgCl_2$, 500 μM ATP (1 x 10^6 cpm [^{32}γP]ATP, 20 μg phosphatidylserine, 2 μg diolein and 25 μl (15 μg total protein) of soluble protein Kinase C (RAMWANI et al, 1989). The reaction was stopped by the addition of 3.0 ml of 10% TCA and filtered through an Amicon filter (GF/C filters).
[≠]means and standard deviations from 3 experiments

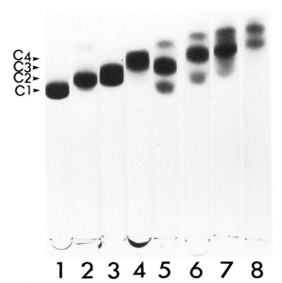

Fig 2   Alkaline-Urea Gels of C-1 → C-4 from MBP and corresponding phosphorylated components. Lanes 1 - 4, C-1 → C-4; lanes 5 - 6, C-1 → C-4 after phosphorylation by protein Kinase C from brain.

Table 2. The relative proportions of a-helix, b-structure, random structure and turns in charge isomers of human myelin basic protein

Protein	Relative Proportion of the Secondary Structures[*]			
	$f\alpha$	$f\beta$	f_r	f_t
C1	0	0.13±0.01	0.64±0.02	0.23±0.02
C2	0	0.19	0.57	0.24
C3	0	0.17	0.59	0.24
C4	0	0.24±.05	0.57±0.06	0.19±0.02

$f\alpha$ = proportion of α helix

$f\beta$ = proportion of β-structure

f_r = proportion of random

f_t = proportion of turns.

[*]The relative proportions of secondary structure were obtained from an analysis of data points at 1 nm intervals between 190 - 240 nm by the least square method. The sum of the fractions of each structure was constrained to add up to 1.0. The reference data were obtained from 15 water soluble proteins provided by Yang (23). The values for C-1 and C-4 are the means and standard errors of the mean from 6 independent preparations of the components. The values for C-2 and C-3 are single determinations from a single set of spectra. However, they are in good agreement with two additional sets of spectra.

C-4 represent the means and standard errors for six independent preparations of components. Although those for C-2 and C-3 are from a single set of spectra they are in good agreement with those from two additional sets of spectra. Phosphorylation of the components increased the proportion of β-structure in all cases. Thus the proportion of β-structure in C-1 increased from 0.13±0.01 - 0.37±0.05. Similar increases were observed in C-2, C-3 while C-4 increased from 0.24±0.05 - 0.41±0.04 (Table 3). Since C-1 showed the largest increase in β-structure it was treated with acid phosphatase for 30 min, to dephosphorylate it to determine if the spectral changes we observed were reversible. Only 50% of the [^{32}P]PO$_4$ transferred to C-1 could be removed even after prolonged digestion (24 h), and no change in the proportion of β-structure was found (Table 4). We concluded that the PO$_4$ not accessible to the enzyme was in a highly structured site. In order to identify the protected site, the phosphorylated C-1 was treated with endoproteinase Lys C after the acid phosphatase digestion. The peptides were resolved by HPLC and the composition of the single radioactive peptide was determined which corresponded to residues 5-13 of the human sequence (Arg-Pro-Ser-Gln-Arg-His-Gly-Ser-Lys). Further digestion of this peptide with trypsin and resolution of the mixture on HPLC allowed us to demonstrate that the Ser residue at position 7 was the principal phosphorylated amino acid. Examination of this peptide (Fig 3) shows that the Ser residue phosphorylated is flanked by Arg Pro on the left and by Gln Arg on the right. By neutralizing the

Table 3. Relative proportions of α-helix, β-structure, random structure and turns in charge isomers of human myelin basic protein after phosphorylation

Charge Isomer	Relative proportions of the Secondary Structures[*]			
	fα	fβ	f_r	f_t
C1	0	0.37±0.05	0.43±0.08	0.20±0.03
C2	0	0.40	0.40	0.20
C3	0	0.39	0.41	0.20
C4	0	0.41±0.04	0.40±0.002	0.19±0.01

[*] See legend Table 2

Table 4. The relative proportions of a-helix, b-structure, random structure and turns of Component 1 from human MBP

	Relative proportions of the Secondary Structures[†]			
Component 1	fα	fβ	f_r	f_t
Phosphorylated[*]	0	0.45	0.38	0.17
Acid Phosphatase (1h)	0	0.38	0.43	0.20

[*]Both phosphorylated and nonphosphorylated C-1 were dissolved in 0.1M sodium acetate buffer pH 4.8 for these experiments.
† See legend Table I for details of phosphorylation experiments.

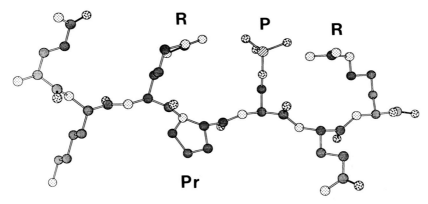

Fig 3   Model of Phosphorylated Site of Peptide 5-13 of Human MBP Sequence in b-Structure

Shaded balls   ⬤   represent carbon atoms

Stippled balls   ⬤   represent nitrogen atoms

Spotted balls   ⬤   represent oxygen atoms
P -   represents phosphorylated Ser residue
Pr -   proline ring
R -   Arg
Q -   glutamine is shown below plane of the peptide.
The guanidino group of both Arg residues is shown in close proximity to the phosphate on Ser 7.

two positive charges on the Arg residues 5, 9, an apolar segment is generated. From the molecular model of this peptide constructed in β-conformation it can ben seen that the guanidyl groups of the two Arg residues approach each other which can interact with the negatively charged phosphate group generating a symmetrical, highly stable structure. The Pro residue at position 6 would help to stabilize the structure possibly by being involved in a bend. Therefore, the lack of acid phosphatase sensitivity is due to the protected conformation of this phosphorylated peptide. Furthermore, this site appears to a "critical" site, since the stability of the β-structure of the molecule depends largely on the β-conformation at this site (RAMWANI and MOSCARELLO, unpublished).

GTP Binding and ADP-ribosylation

Protein Kinase C has been demonstrated in myelin (SCHULZ *et al, 1988*). Along with phospholipase-C, phosphatidylinositol bisphosphate, Ca^{++}, phosphatidylserine, diacylglycerol, all the

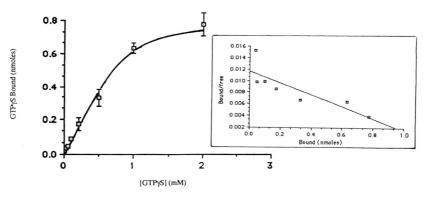

Fig 4   Binding of GTPgS to Component 1 of Human MBP.
Maximum binding was obtained at a GTPγS concentration of 1 mM; corresponding to a nucleotide to protein ratio of 1:2. Inset: Scatchard plot of the binding of GTPγS to MBP. The estimated value for B_{max} is 0.98±0.02 nmoles in the presence of 1.34 nmoles MBP (25 μg) which corresponds to a mole ratio of nucleotide to protein 0.74 to 1. The K_D obtained by Scatchard plot is 0.82±0.16 mM. B_{max} is defined as the maximum binding of MBP for GTPγS which is the X-intercept of the Scatchard plot. The K_D is defined as the dissociation constant of MBP for GTPγS which is equal to the negative reciprocal of the slope.

components of a signal transduction system are present except a G protein. In this section evidence is presented showing that MBP can bind GTP at a specific site and that it can be ADP-ribosylated by Cholera toxin, fulfilling two of three essential criteria by which a "G" protein is identified. That of GTPase activity in MBP has not been fulfilled yet although myelin has been shown to have GTPase activity.

To study the binding of GTP to C-1 of MBP, a non hydrolysable analogue, GTPγS, labelled with [^{35}S] was used (CHAN *et al*, 1988). These data are shown in Fig 4. Maximum binding was observed at 1.0 mM GTPγS, corresponding to a nucleotide to protein ratio of 1:2. In competition experiments both GppNHp and GTPγS were able to compete for azido GTP labelling of MBP (Fig 5). GppNHp is another non-hydrolysable analogue of GTP but is less effective in competing out azido GTP binding. In order to identify the GTP binding site, MBP was

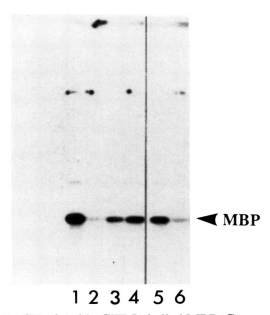

◀ MBP

1 2 3 4 5 6

Fig 5   SDS-PAGE of Azido GTP Labelled MBP. Component 1 was labelled with [^{32}P]-Azido GTP under different conditions. Lane 1, azido GTP labelled protein; lane 2, azido GTP labelling of C-1 in the presence of GTPγS; lane 3, in the presence of GTP; lane 4, in the presence of GDP; lane 5, in the presence of ATP; lane 6, in the presence of azido GTP but not irradiated.

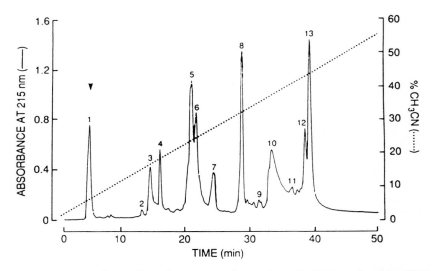

Fig 6   HPLC profile of endoproteinase Lys C digest of azido-GTP
         bound MBP. MBP (0.5 mg) was photolabelled with azido-
         GTP (CHAN *et al*, 1988). The azido-GTP labelled MBP was
         then digested by endoproteinase Lys C yielding 13 peptides.
         Among these 13 peptides, only peptide #1 was radioactive
         (shown by an arrow).

reacted with the photo-affinity label, 8-azido GTP [γ^{32}P]. The proteinase
Lys C digest was resolved on reversed phase HPLC, which yielded a
single radioactive peptide (Fig 6). Amino acid analysis of this peptide
gave the composition Ala, Ser, Glu, Lys in the ratio 1.0/1.24/0.62/0.83.
This composition corresponds to the N-terminal peptide Ac-Ala-Ser-Gln-
Lys. The low recovery of Gln suggested that azido GTP bound to this
amino acid. Further support for the conclusion that Gln was the residue
to which GTP was bound was obtained by carboxy peptidase S, digestion
of the labelled peptide. Only Lys was released, suggesting that
modification of the Gln residue prevented further digestion. From these
data it can be concluded that MBP is a GTP-binding protein. Further data
is required, i.e. a demonstration that it contains GTPase activity, to
establish that it may function in the myelin sheath in a signal transducing
system.

      ADP-Ribosylation of C-1, C-2, C-3 and C-8 of MBP was carried
out in the presence of Cholera toxin and [^{32}P] NAD (BOULIAS and
MOSCARELLO, 1989). The SDS-PAGE of this reaction is shown in Fig
7. Whereas C-1, C-2 and C-3 were all ADP-ribosylated, C-8 was not,
highlighting the difference in behaviour of the various components. A

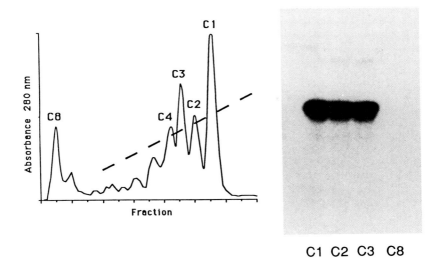

C1 C2 C3 C8

Fig 7   ADP-Ribosylation of Components of Human MBP with
Cholera Toxin. After ADP-ribosylation with [32P]-NAD, the
protein was run on SDS-PAGE and exposed to X-ray film.
The right hand panel of Fig 7 shows the radioautograph. C-1,
C-2 and C-3 were ADP-ribosylated while C-8 was not. The
left hand panel shows the resolution of components of human
MBP by CM52 cation exchange chromatography.

time course of incubation showed that C-1, C-2 and C-3 were ADP-
ribosylated, reaching a maximum in 90 min. C-8 on the other hand was
not ADP-ribosylated in a time-dependent manner. Quantitation of the
amount of ADP-ribose incorporated is shown in Table 5. C-1, C-2 and
C-3 each incorporated about 1 mole ADP-ribose/mole protein while C-8
only incorporated 0.11 moles. Sensitivity of the ADP-ribosylated C-1 to
hydroxylamine suggested that ADP-ribosylation occurred at an Arg
residue. From these studies we concluded that MBP can be ADP-
ribosylated by Cholera toxin probably on an arginyl residue.
Identification of the site to which ADP-ribose binds is underway by
isolating ADP-ribosylated peptides from Lys C digest.

From the data presented so far it is clear that the various
components of MBP are (i) conformationally different in that they contain
different amounts of β-structure; (ii) they can be phosphorylated to
different extents in the order C-1 < C-2 < C-3 < C-4;   (iii)

Table 5. The specific activities of myelin basic protein components after ADP-ribosylation

MBP Component	Total protein	Total activity	Specific activity
	nmoles	nmoles of ADP-R bound	moles ADP-R/ mole protein
C-1	0.111	0.131	1.18
C-2	0.111	0.121	1.09
C-3	0.087	0.083	1.05
C-8	0.108	0.012	0.11

C-1, C-2, C-3 and C-8 were ADP-ribosylated with [^{32}P] NAD in the presence of Cholera Toxin for 90 min. The moles of ADP-ribose transferred were computed from the specific activity of the [^{32}P] NAD. The protein was determined by amino acid analyses.

phosphorylation affects the secondary structure by increasing the amount of β-structure in the order C-1 > C-2 > C-3 > C-4; (iv) the phosphate group at Ser 7 is not accessible to hydrolysis by acid phosphatase; (v) C-1 binds azido GTP at a single site at Gln 3 of the human sequence; (vi) C-1, C-2 and C-3 can be ADP-ribosylated while C-8 cannot. All the studies mentioned above involve the addition of a negatively charged phosphoryl group to the protein rendering it less cationic. Modification of MBP with neutral sugar has been observed also which has interesting and different effects on the interaction of the protein with a lipid bilayer i.e. whereas phosphorylation decreases interaction, glycosylation enhances the interaction.

Glycosylation of MBP

Glycosylation of bovine MBP was demonstrated first by HAGOPIAN and EYLAR in 1969. They were able to transfer N-acetyl-D-galactosamine from UDP-N-acetyl-D-galactosamine to Thr 98 of the bovine sequence with a galactosaminyl transferase from bovine submaxillary gland. With human MBP we were able to show that both Thr 95 and Thr 98 were glycosylated in the presence of a galactosaminyl transferase from porcine submaxillary gland (CRUZ and MOSCARELLO, 1983; CRUZ et al, 1984). Since two sites were glycosylated we wanted to know if the order of addition was random or directed. The positions of both Thr 95 and 98 in the proton NMR spectra of MBP have been established by Mendz et al, 1983. With this information we were able to study the proton NMR spectra of MBP glycosylated with 1.1 mol GALNAC/mol protein and 1.5 mol GALNAC/mol protein. The data are shown in Fig 8. The resonances corresponding to Thr 95 and 98 can be seen readily in the non-glycosylated sample (A, in the panel). After addition of 1.1 mol GALNAC/mol MBP the resonances corresponding to Thr 95 have shifted and are no longer visible. After the addition of 1.5 mol GALNAC/mol MBP the resonances corresponding to Thr 98 are also shifted. These data establish the order of glycosylation as being sequential i.e. Thr 95 is glycosylated first followed by Thr 98. The spectra also demonstrate that other resonances are also affected. Thus the Ala β and Val γ envelopes situated at 1.42 and 1.46 ppm respectively are also affected. Whereas these resonances show a wide chemical shift dispersion in the unglycosylated protein, these resonances coalesce with increasing glycosylation indicative of similar chemical environments for these resonances (PERSAUD et al, 1988). We interpreted this to suggest changes in secondary structure throughout the molecule as the result of glycosylation. An examination of the sequence of the human MBP shows that all three Val residues are near the glycosylation site at positions 86, 87, 94. However, the Ala residues are spread throughout the molecule from the N-terminus to the C-terminus. Therefore the coalescences observed in the proton NMR spectra of the Ala β and Val γ protons suggests the changes in secondary structure affect the entire molecule.

The interaction of glycosylated MBP with lipid bilayers was studied by electron spin resonance after chemically introducing a spin label on the GALNAC. To do this, MBP was glycosylated with 0.85 moles GALNAC/mol protein so that only Thr 95 was glycosylated. The hydroxyl group of carbon six of the GALNAC was oxidized with galactose oxidase and complexed with a spin label TEMPOAMINE as shown in Fig 9 (PERSAUD et al, 1989). Interaction of this spin labelled-glycosylated MBP with various lipids demonstrated motional restriction of the probe which we attributed to penetration part way into the lipid bilayer in both gel and liquid crystalline phases. The ability of segments of the protein to penetrate into the lipid bilayer was confirmed by Lys C digestion of the vesicle-bound protein followed by separation on a C:18 μ Bondapak reversed phase column. The pattern obtained for non-glycosylated and glycosylated MBP in solution are shown in Fig 10 A and B respectively. The peptide maps are similar, showing extensive digestion by the proteinase, although some differences can be seen. The peptide eluting at 25 min contained 80% of the [14C]-labelled GALNAC. This peptide was collected and further purified by HPLC. It was identified as peptide 92-105 which contained the major glycosylation site. Hydrolysis of this peptide in 5.7 N HCl for 4 h at 100° followed by amino acid analysis for amino sugar demonstrated that all the [14C] was recovered in galatosamine.

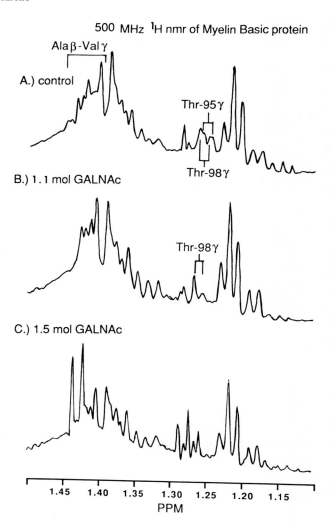

Fig 8   Proton (500 mHz) Spectra of Non Glycosylated and
        Glycosylated MBP.
        A.   Control - Non Glycosylated MBP.
        B.   Glycosylated MBP with 1.1 mol [14C]GALNAC/mol
             MBP. The Thr 95 resonances are shifted.
        C.   Glycosylated MBP with 1.5 mol [14C]GALNAC/mol
             MBP. Both Thr 95 and Thr 98 resonances are shifted.

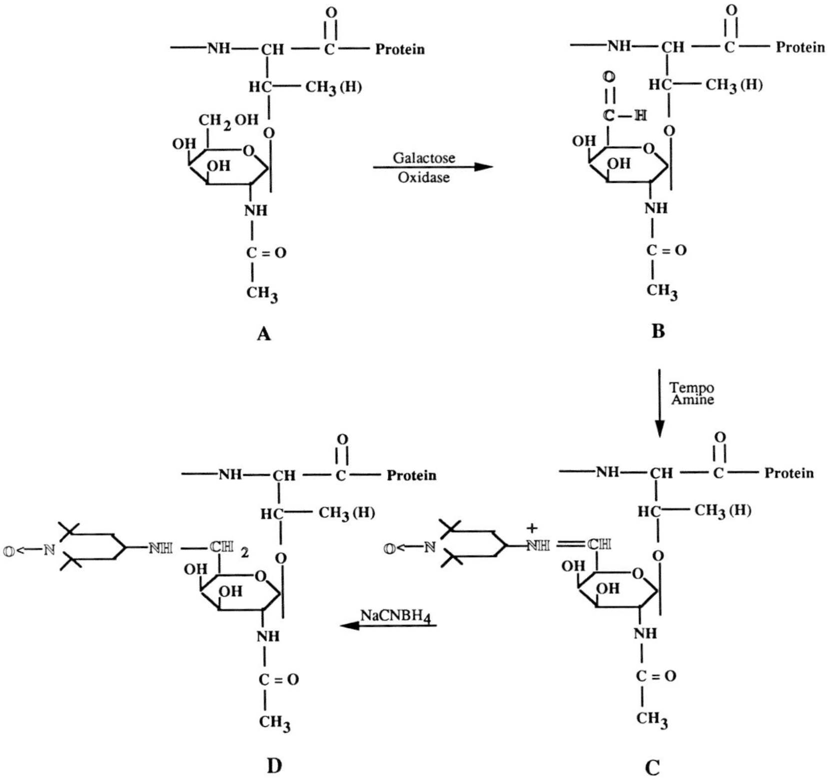

Fig 9   Spin Labelling of [14C]-GALNAC Labelled MBP.
An outline of the combined enzymatic and chemical method of
spin labelling glycosylated basic protein (A). The first step
involved the formation of an aldehyde by oxidation of the
hydroxyl at C-6 with the enzyme galactose oxidase (B).
Reaction with tempoamine generated the imine adduct (C).
Reduction with cyanoborohydride produced the stable spin
labelled protein (D).

When similar experiments were carried out with the non-
glycosylated and glycosylated proteins in lipid vesicles
(dipalmitoylphosphatidylglycerol, DPPG), we obtained the profiles
shown in Fig 10 C & D. Although considerable digestion was obtained
when non glycosylated MBP (C), was incorporated into DPPG the
peptide map was significantly different from that obtained for the non-
glycosylated MBP in solution (A), demonstrating that some sites
susceptible to Lys C were protected by the lipid. When the glycosylated

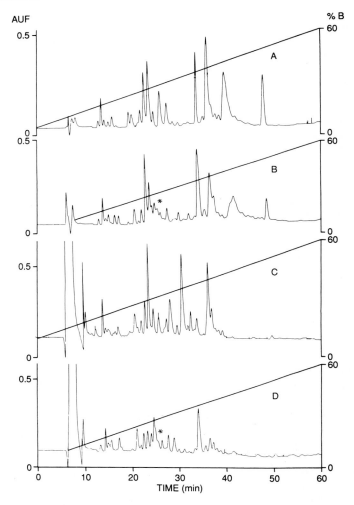

Fig 10   HPLC Profile of Endoproteinase Lys C Digest of Non
          Glycosylated and Glycosyalted MBP with [14C]-GALNAC.
          A. Digest of MBP in solution
          B. Digest of [14C]-GALNAC, glycosylated MBP
          C. Digest of MBP in lipid vesicles consisting of 92.2%
              phosphatidylcholine and 7.8% phosphatidylserine
          D. Digest of [14C]-GALNAC, Glycosylated MBP in lipid
              vesicles consisting of 92.2% phosphatidylcholine and
              7.8% phosphatidylserine.

MBP was incorporated into lipid vesicles, the peptide map was very different from any of the others (D), demonstrating that few Lys C sites were available to the enzyme. When the glycosylated peptide was isolated from this digest it accounted for, less than 10% of this peptide present in MBP. However the small number of peptides released by Lys C suggests that glycosylation at Thr 95 has affected the interaction of the entire molecule with the lipid probably as a result of changes in secondary structure. We are currently studying the secondary structure of the glycosylated protein to define it more accurately. It probably reflects a considerable increase in β-structure which has been documented for MBP in lipid vesicles by FOURIER TRANSFORM INFRA RED recently (SUREWICZ *et al,* 1987). The data presented here for the glycosylated MBP, support the data on phosphorylation presented earlier demonstrating that post-translational modifications have important and far reaching effects on the folded structure of MBP and its interaction with lipids.

The Presence of Citrulline in MBP

When MBP is fractionated on CM-52 columns to isolate the components a significant amount of material (25-30%) of adult human MBP fails to bind to the column (Fig 7) because it is much less cationic than C-1. Amino acid analyses of this material were consistent with its identity as MBP except that the amount of Arg recovered was very low (Table 6) i.e. only about 13 instead of 19 per mole. Some years back we reported that some myelin proteins which were poorly characterized at the time contained significant amounts of citrulline, a known post translational modification of arginine (FINCH *et al* , 1971). Since the deimination of arginine results in loss of the positive charge on the guanidino group, the less cationic nature of C-8 can be explained largely on this basis. Amino acid analyses of several of the components for citrulline are shown in Table 7. C-1, C-2, C-3 contained trace amounts of citrulline only, C-4 had a measurable amount while C-8 contained 5.4 mol/mol protein. Ornithine is included in the citrulline values because it is generated by strong acid hydrolysis of citrulline. Clearly, the amount of citrulline recovered accounted for all the missing arginine.

In order to determine which of the 19 arginine residues were replaced by citrulline, we did the entire amino acid sequence of C-8 after both chemical (cyanogen bromide and BNPS-Skatole) and enzymatic (Cathepsin D and carboxypeptidase S 1) digestions. Citrulline was found replacing arginine at residues 25, 31, 122, 130, 159 and 169 of the human sequence. The replacements were not random but were clustered in the N and C-terminal portions of the molecule. The significance of this distribution will be alluded to later (WOOD & MOSCARELLO, 1989).

Table 6. Amino Acid Composition of Component "C-8" (Residues/100)

For each amino acid analysis, 10 µg protein were hydrolysed in liquid phase with
5.7N HCL at 110° for 24 h. After lyophilization, the amino acid mixture was derivitized
and resolved on a Water's Pico Tag System.

Amino Acid	Isolated from Basic Protein	Basic Protein 18.5 KDa	Isolated from Lipophilin
ASX[a]	7.3 ± 0.64	6.5	6.5
THR	5.4 ± 0.26	4.7	5.5
SER	10.9 ± 0.5	11.2	11.4
GLX[b]	8.0 ± 0.58	5.3*	7.2
PRO	8.0 ± 0.49	7.1	10.0
GLY	16.4 ± 0.61	15.3	16.3
ALA	7.9 ± 0.43	7.1	7.7
VAL	2.2 ± 0.18	2.4	1.9
1/2 CYS	-	-	-
MET	0.8 ± 0.38	1.2	0.33
ILEU	2.1 ± 0.18	2.4	1.7
LEU	4.9 ± 0.33	4.7	4.4
TYR	2.4 ± 0.14	2.4	2.0
PHE	4.9 ± 0.36	5.3	4.6
LYS	6.3 ± 0.78	7.1	6.4
HIS	6.0 ± 0.45	5.9	6.1
ARG	6.9 ± 0.68	11.2*	8.0
TRP[‡]	+	1.0	

*Amino acids considered different from known composition
The mean and standard deviations were derived from 6 amino acid analyses, of 6
independent samples.
‡TRP was detected by intrinsic fluorescence
ASX[a] = ASP + ASN
GLX[b] = GLU + GLN

TABLE 7. Citrulline Analyses on Charge Isomers from Myelin Basic Protein

The various charge isomers were separated on CM-52 columns at pH 10.6 as
described in Methods. After hydrolysis in 5.7 N HCl, at 110° for 24 h the hydrolysates
were analyzed on the Beckman physiological system (Beckman 7300). The total amount of
citrulline was the sum of citrulline + ornithine.

COMPONENT	residues/100 CITRULLINE	ORNITHINE	TOTAL
C-1	N.D*	N.D*	-
C-2	0.13	0.13	0.26
C-3	0.15	0.20	0.35
C-4	0.28	0.40	0.68
"C-8"	3.90	1.5	5.40

*N.D.- not detected

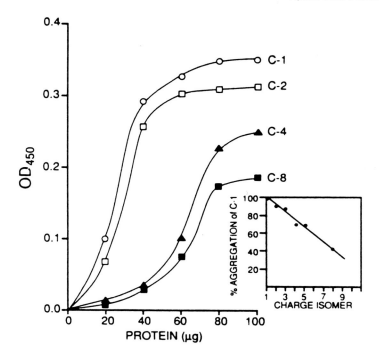

Fig 11   Vesicle Aggregation of Components from Human MBP in Lipid Vesicles Consisting of 92.2% Phosphatidylcholine and 7.8% Phosphatidylserine. Vesicle aggregation was measured at 450 nm, maintaining the amount of lipid constant and increasing the amount of protein. The inset shows the linear relationship between % aggregation of C-1 and charge isomers.

Some insight into the functional significance of the presence of citrulline has been obtained and will be mentioned briefly. The loss of positive charge affects the ability of the protein to interact with lipids. Thus in lipid vesicles consisting of 92.2 mols % phosphatidyl-choline and 7.8 mol % of phosphatidylserine, C-8 was much less effective at inducing vesicle aggregation than C-1, C-2 or C-4 (Fig 11). On the other hand when vesicles were prepared of phosphatidylcholine only containing lipophilin C-8 was able to induce good vesicle aggregation while C-1, C-2 and C-4 failed to induce aggregation (Fig 12). This data suggested to us that C-8 had a particular affinity for lipophilin since the presence of the latter was essential for vesicle aggregation. Further evidence of this affinity was demonstrated in the close association between lipophilin and a fraction of MBP. When lipophilin is isolated by LH-20 chromatogaphy in

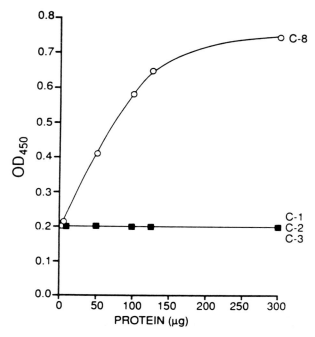

Fig 12   Vesicle Aggregation of Components from Human MBP in Phosphatidylcholine Vesicles Containing 50% (w/w) of Lipophilin (human PLP).

acidified chloroform/methanol a small amount of MBP remains firmly associated with it. This MBP can be readily removed by acetic acid extraction of lyophilized lipophilin. When run on CM-52 columns it behaves like C-8 and the amino acid composition is similar to C-8, notably in the low values of arginine (Table 6). Further studies on this material are necessary to establish the sites of the arginine replacements.

Our interest in this C-8 material has been stimulated further by the observation that MBP isolated from the brains of human infants from 5 days to 15 months of age is all C-8 by CM-52 cation exchange chromatography. None of the other components have been found up to the age of 15 months. Amino acid analyses of this C-8 material demonstrated that the expected amount of citrulline was present. These data are suggestive of a "fetal" type MBP although this is purely speculative.

The presence of citrulline at these distinct sites can be explained by one of several possibilities; (a) the conformation of the protein may be

such that only arginines at positions 25, 31, 122, 130, 159 and 169 are accessible to the peptidylarginine deiminase, an enzyme in brain which is known to convert arginine in peptide bond to citrulline in peptide bond;
 (b) the genetic code contains information which is translated through the amino acid sequence directing the deimination of specific arginine residues. From an examination of the DNA sequence (KALMHOLZ et al, 1986), all the Arg codons corresponding to sites of arginine replacements are either AGA or AGG. The amino acid coded for on either side of the Arg is either apolar or hydrophobic except the C-terminal amino acid which is Arg. Since this residue contains one positive charge and one negative charge it is in fact neutral and can be considered apolar. The mechanism through which this arginine to citrulline replacement is regulated is not understood. Although the above mentioned comments are purely speculative, they provide the basis for several interesting experiments at the molecular biological level.

TO SUMMARIZE

MBP undergoes a large number of post translational modifications by both charge and non charged groups (Fig 13). These generate a family of microheteromers which influences the mechanism by which the protein interacts in a lipid bilayer on a charge basis. On the other hand, some of the modifications we have discussed affect the secondary structure of the protein primarily which then affects its ability to interact with lipids. Since myelin contains several enzymes, the possibility that these or similar changes actually occur in situ must be considered highly probable, imparting to myelin a continuously changing structure, in some cases analogous to a "breathing motion". In addition, a continuously changing structure of MBP, can generate a changing panorama of epitopes which would elicit a changing population of sensitized cells. This concept of different antigenic determinants may have implications towards an understanding of human disease multiple sclerosis. Thus in an acute phase of the disease, sensitized cells are generated to a particular epitope which the organism learns to handle. However, a subsequent attack may involve a different epitope, generated by one of the mechanisms mentioned above which would generate a different population of sensitized cells. In studying MS tissue sensitivity to the original epitope may decrease markedly after one or two attacks making correlations between exacerbation and exposure of specific antigenic determinants difficult, especially when assaying for epitopes generated by the linear sequence of amino acids.

POSITIONS OF KNOWN POST-TRANSLATIONAL MODIFICATIONS ON HUMAN MYELIN BASIC PROTEIN

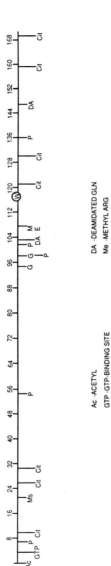

Ac -ACETYL
GTP -GTP-BINDING SITE
Cit -CITRULLINE (DEIMINATION OF ARG)
P -PHOSPHATE
G -N-ACETYL-D-GALACTOSAMINE

DA -DEAMIDATED GLN
Me -METHYL ARG
Ms -METHIONINE SULFOXIDE
W -TRYPTOPHAN

Fig 13   Post Translational Modifications of MBP. Citrulline at position
9 is tentative.   Thr 98 can be either glycosylated or
phosphorylated. Phosphorylation at Ser 54 is tentative.

REFERENCES

Boggs JM, Moscarello MA, Papahadjopoulos D (1982). Structural organization of myelin-role of lipid-protein interactions determined in model membranes, in lipid-protein interactions. Vol. 2, Jost, P.C. and Griffith, O.H. ed. Academic Press N.Y. pp 1-51.

Boulias C, Moscarello MA (1989). ADP-ribosylation of charge isomers of myelin basic protein. Submitted.

Chan CK, Ramwani J, Moscarello MA (1988). Myelin basic protein binds GTP at a single site in the N-terminus. Biochem. Biophys Res. Comm. 152 : 1468-1473.

Chang TC, Wu CCS, Yang JT (1978). Circular dichroic analysis of protein conformation: inclusion of the β-turns. Analytical Biochemistry 91:13-31.

Cheifetz S, Moscarello MA (1985). Effect of bovine charge microheterogeneity on protein-induced aggregation of unilamellar vesicles containing a mixture of acidic and neutral phospholipids. Biochemistry 24 : 1909-1914.

Cheifetz S, Boggs JM, Moscarello MA (1985). Increase in vesicle permeability mediated by myelin basic protein: effect of phosphorylation of basic protein. Biochemistry 24: 5170-5175.

Cruz TF, Moscarello MA (1983). Identification of the major sites of enzymic glycosylation of myelin basic protein. Biochim et Biophys Acta 760 : 403-410.

Cruz TF, Wood DD, Moscarello, MA (1984). Identification of Thr 95 as the major site of glycosylation in normal human myelin basic protein. Biochem J. 220 : 849-852.

Deibler GE, Martenson RE (1973). Chromatographic fractionation of myelin basic protein. J. Biol. Chem. 248 : 2392-2396.

Finch PR, Wood DD, Moscarello MA (1971). The presence of citrulline in a myelin protein fraction. Febs Letts 15 : 145-148.

Hagopian A, Eylar EH (1969). Glycoprotein biosynthesis. The purification and characterization of a polypeptide-n-acetylgalacto-saminyl transferase from bovine submaxillary glands. Arch. Biochem and Biophys 129 : 515-524.

Kalmholz J, de Fera F, Puckett C, Lazzarini R (1986). Identification of three forms of human myelin basic protein by cDNA cloning. Proc. Nat. Acad. Sci (USA) 83 : 4962-4966.

Martenson RE, Deibler GE, Kies MW (1969). Microheterogeneity of guinea pig myelin basic protein. J. Biol. Chem. 244: 4261-4267.

Mendz GL, Moore WJ, Martenson RE (1983). NMR studies on myelin basic protein. VIII. Complete assignment of the threonine residues by proton NMR of proteins from five species. Biochim et Biophys Acta 742 : 215-223.

Miyamoto E, Kakiuchi S (1974). In vitro and in vivo phosphorylation of myelin basic protein by exogenous and endogenous adenosine 3'5' monophosphate dependent protein kinases in brain. J. Biol. Chem. 249: 2769-2777.

Murray N, Steck AJ (1984). Impulse conduction regulates myelin basic protein phosphorylation in rat optic nerve. J. Neurochem 43 : 243-248.

Norton WT, Cammer W (1984). Isolation and characterization of myelin, in Myelin. P. Morell, editor, Plenum Press N.Y. p. 165.

Persaud R, Boggs JM, Wood DD, Moscarello MA (1989). The interaction of glycosylated human myelin basic protein with lipid bilayers. Biochemistry (in press).

Persaud R, Fraser P, Wood DD, Moscarello MA (1988). The glycosylation of human myelin basic protein at Thr 95 and 98 occurs sequentially. Biochim et Biophys Acta 966 : 357-361.

Ramwani J, Epand RM, Moscarello MA (1989). The secondary structure of charge isomers of myelin basic protein before and after phosphorylation. Biochemistry, in press.

Rumsby MG (1987). Structural organization and stability of central nervous system myelin, in a multidisciplinary approach to myelin diseases. Crescenzi, G.S. ed. Nato Asi Series. Series A, Life Sciences 142: 111-132.

Schulz P, Cruz TF, Moscarello MA (1988). Endogenous phosphorylation of basic protein in myelin of varying degrees of compaction. Biochemistry 27 : 7793-7799.

Surewicz W, Moscarello MA, Mantsch H (1987). Fourier transform infrared spectroscopic investigation of the interaction between myelin basic protein and dimyristoylphosphatidylglycerol bilayers. Biochemistry 26 : 3881-3886.

Wood D.D, Moscarello M. (1989). The Isolation, characterization and lipid-aggregating properties of a citrulline containing myelin basic protein. J. Biol. Chem. 264:5121-5127.

Dynamic Interactions of Myelin Proteins, pages 49–79
© 1990 Alan R. Liss, Inc.

THE IMMUNOGLOBULIN GENE SUPERFAMILY AND MYELINATION

Richard H. Quarles, Jeffrey A. Hammer and
Bruce D. Trapp

NINDS, NIH, Bethesda, MD 20892 (R.H.Q.&
J.A.H.), and Department of Neurology, The Johns
Hopkins University School of Medicine,
Baltimore, MD 21205 (B.D.T.)

INTRODUCTION

The immunoglobulin gene superfamily is a large group
of proteins with amino acid sequence homologies that is
believed to have arisen during evolution from a common
ancestral protein (reviewed in Williams, 1984; 1987).
Members of the family share one or more structures called
immunoglobulin (Ig) homology units (or Ig-like domains)
composed of sequences of about 100 amino acids usually
containing a centrally placed disulphide bridge that helps
to stabilize a series of anti-parallel ß-strands into the
so-called antibody fold. Most proteins involved in the
functioning of the immune system, including the antibodies
themselves, are members of the family. However, in recent
years it has become apparent that the nervous system also
contains proteins in this family that are involved in
cell-cell interactions (Williams, 1987). The structures
of some representative members of the family in the
immune system are shown in Figure 1. They range from
simple molecules with one Ig-like domain such as Thy-1 at
the left of the figure to much more complex molecules with
numerous domains such as the antibody shown at the far
right. The polyimmunoglobulin receptor is included in the
figure because its overall structure, with five Ig-like
domains linearly arranged in a single polypeptide chain
and a relatively large, cytoplasmic, C-terminal tail, is
very similar to some neural members of the family that
will be considered in more detail below. A property of

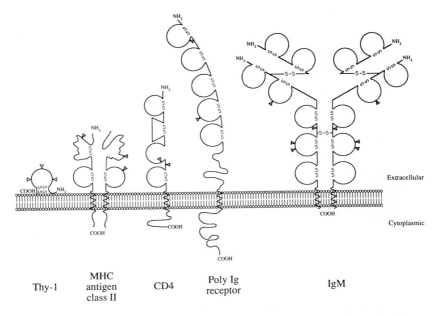

Figure 1. Examples of immune system glycoproteins in the immunoglobulin gene superfamily. Each circular structure closed by a disulfide bond represents a single Ig-like domain. Structures from Williams (1984; 1985).

members of this family that is relevant to their function in cell-cell interactions is that they often bind to other Ig-like proteins. For example, among the molecules shown in Fig. 1, the class II major histocompatibility antigen binds to the CD4 protein during T cell activation (Gay et al, 1987), and the polyimmunoglobulin receptor binds IgM and IgA during the transport of antibodies across epithelial cells (Mostov et al, 1984).

The principal subject of this chapter is the involvement of neural proteins of the immunoglobulin superfamily in the process of myelination. Clearly myelination involves cell-cell interactions; the interaction of oligodendrocytes with neuronal axons in the CNS and the interaction of Schwann cells with axons in the PNS. Figure 2 shows five neural members of the immunoglobulin gene superfamily. Thy-1 is included again

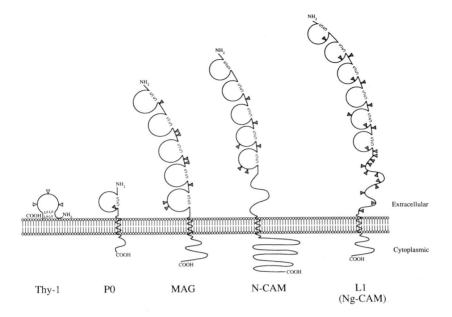

Figure 2. Examples of neural glycoproteins in the immunoglobulin gene superfamily. Each of these neural proteins has been shown to be a member of the immunoglobulin superfamily based on amino acid sequence homologies: Thy-1 (Williams and Gagnon, 1982), P0 (Lemke and Axel, 1985; Uyemura et al, 1987), MAG (Arquint et al, 1987; Lai et al, 1987; Salzer et al, 1987), N-CAM (Cunningham et al, 1987; Barthels et al, 1987); L1 (Moos et al, 1988).

since it is expressed by cells in both the immune and nervous systems. The P0 glycoprotein of peripheral nervous system myelin similarly has just one Ig-like domain but is specific for the nervous system. The three proteins to the right of Figure 2 with five or six Ig-like domains on a single polypeptide chain have been shown to be involved in neuron-neuron and/or neuron-glia interactions. Perhaps the most extensively studied is neural cell adhesion molecule (N-CAM) which is believed to function in cell adhesion by homophilic binding; i.e. N-CAM molecules on one cell bind to other N-CAM molecules on

an adjacent cell. The structure and function of N-CAM has
been reviewed in detail elsewhere (Edelman, 1986; 1987)
and will only be discussed here in the context of
myelination. All of the neural members of the family
shown in Figure 2 are present and have been studied
extensively in mammals. However, neural proteins in the
immunoglobulin gene superfamily that are involved in cell-
cell interactions have also been identified in insects
(Harrelson and Goodman, 1988) adding strength to the
hypothesis that the family arose during evolution from
ancestral molecules involved in cell-cell interactions,
and that the immune system itself is a later very
sophisticated extension of the family. The emphasis in
this chapter will be placed on P0 glycoprotein and the
myelin-associated glycoprotein (MAG) which are nervous
system specific and appear to function primarily in
myelination. However, N-CAM and L1 (Ng-CAM) are also
expressed by myelin-forming cells and are likely to be
important for myelination in addition to other neural cell
interactions.

P0 GLYCOPROTEIN

     The P0 glycoprotein is the major protein of
peripheral nerve myelin, accounting for more than 50% of
the total protein in purified myelin. The complete amino
acid sequence of rat P0 was determined from a cDNA (Lemke
and Axel, 1985) and that of bovine P0 by automatic Edman
degradation of peptide fragments (Sakomoto et al, 1987).
The sequence reveals a single membrane spanning domain
separating a 68 amino acid intracellular domain from a 124
amino acid extracellular domain with significant amino
acid similarities to variable region folds of immunoglobulins and other members of the immunoglobulin gene
superfamily (Lai et al, 1987; Lai et al, 1988; Lemke et
al, 1988; Uyemura et al, 1987). The extracellular portion
of the molecule carries all the essential features of
prototypical Ig domains including two cysteine residues
separated by 77 amino acids as well as reiterated
stretches of alternating hydrophobic amino acids. It has
long been thought from histochemical and surface probe
studies (reviewed in Quarles, 1979) that part of the P0
molecule is in the intraperiod line of PNS myelin and may
play a role in stabilizing the apposition of extracellular
membrane surfaces. Since members of the immunoglobulin

superfamily often bind to other members of the family or
exhibit homophilic binding, the likelihood that this is
the case is increased. Lemke and Axel (1985) suggested
that it might do so by homophilic binding similarly to the
functioning of N-CAM, although in the case of P0 it would
be binding of P0 molecules in one layer of the myelin
spiral to P0 molecules in adjacent layers rather than to
molecules on separate cells (Figure 3).

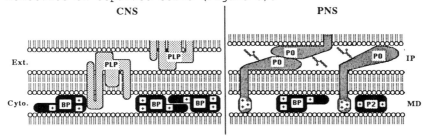

Figure 3. Diagrammatic representation of current concepts
of the molecular organization of compact CNS and PNS
myelin. Apposition of the extracellular (Ext.) surfaces
of the oligodendrocyte or Schwann cell surface membranes
form the intraperiod (IP) line, while the cytoplasmic
(Cyto.) surfaces fuse to form the major dense (MD) line.
BP, myelin basic protein; PLP, proteolipid protein; P0, P0
glycoprotein. Ig-like domains of P0 may interact with
each other to stabilize the intraperiod line of PNS myelin
as represented at the left of the PNS diagram. P0 is not
in CNS myelin, and extracellular domains of PLP probably
stabilize the intraperiod line in the CNS. The cytoplasmic
domain of P0 is positively charged and may help stabilize
the major dense line of PNS myelin together with the
positively charged BP and P2 proteins. MAG is not shown in
the diagrams since it is not present in compact myelin.
Reproduced from Morell et al, 1989 with permission.

MYELIN-ASSOCIATED GLYCOPROTEIN (MAG)

     MAG is a 100 kDa glycoprotein that contains about
one-third by weight carbohydrate and is associated with
myelin in both the central and peripheral nervous systems
(for more detailed review see Quarles, 1988 and in press).
Unlike P0 which is a major component of PNS myelin and
distributed throughout the layered structure of compact
myelin, MAG is a quantitatively minor component of the

whole myelin fraction. Immunocytochemistry has shown that
it is absent from compact myelin and is selectively
localized in the periaxonal membranes of myelin-forming
oligodendrocytes and Schwann cells (Sternberger et al,
1979; Trapp and Quarles, 1982). The periaxonal
localization of MAG provided the first strong suggestion
that MAG could be involved in the interactions between
myelin-forming cells and axons. Stronger evidence that
this is the case will be described below, and the recent
elucidation of the complete amino acid sequence of MAG
from cDNAs (Arquint et al, 1987; Lai et al, 1987; Salzer
et al, 1987) has revealed a number of interesting
properties of the protein that suggest how it may mediate
cell-cell interactions and also suggest that it could play
a very dynamic role in generating the spiraled myelin
sheaths.

As shown in Figure 2, MAG has a single transmembrane
domain separating the glycosylated extracellular part of
the molecule with five Ig-like domains from a relatively
large, cytoplasmic C-terminal tail. For future reference,
the five Ig-like domains are numbered from 1 to 5
beginning at the N-terminus. Each of the Ig-like domains
in MAG shows statistically significant amino acid sequence
homologies with at least one other domain, the strongest
homologies being between domains 3 and 4 which are 45%
identical with many other conservative substitutions (Lai
et al, 1988). There are also many significant homologies
with other family members in both the immune system and
nervous system. Particularly, high alignment scores were
obtained between domains 3, 4 and 5 of MAG and Ig-like
domains of N-CAM. Interestingly, domain 3 of MAG shows a
modest degree of homology with the single Ig-like domain
of P0. The various homologies are reviewed in detail by
Lai et al (1988) who conclude that MAG is prototypical for
the C2 subset of the Ig gene superfamily (Williams, 1987)
that is characterized by sequences characteristic of
variable region domains but with Cys-Cys distances similar
in size or shorter than those that are typical of constant
region domains. This subgroup also includes N-CAM, the
platelet derived growth factor receptor and carcino-
embryonic antigen among other proteins.

The amino acid sequence of rat MAG reveals that
their are eight potential, extracellular,N-linked
glycosylation sites and most appear to be used since the

molecule is about one-third carbohydrate by weight. For
the most part the carbohydrate composition is typical of
N-linked glycoproteins containing mannose, N-acetyl-
glucosamine, galactose, fucose and sialic acid (Quarles et
al, 1983). In MAG isolated from adult rat brain about
two-thirds of the oligosaccharides are tetra- or tri-
antennary, one-third are biantennary, and few or none are
high mannose (Noronha et al, 1989). About one-third of the
oligosaccharides are neutral, and the remainder contain
one or more negative charges (Noronha et al, 1989). Some
of the oligosaccharides are sulfated (Matthieu et al,
1975). A novel carbohydrate structure present on MAG is
defined by the antibody HNK-1 (McGarry et al, 1983; Sato
et al, 1983; Murray and Steck, 1984), although there is
substantial interspecies variation in the amount of this
carbohydrate configuration on MAG; e.g. rat MAG has very
little, whereas human MAG is very rich in the reactive
structure (O'Shannessy et al, 1985). Since HNK-1 was
originally shown to react with human natural killer
lymphocytes (Abo and Balch, 1981), this antibody defines a
carbohydrate epitope that is shared between the nervous
system and the immune system. Thus in addition to the
amino acid sequence homologies with members of the
immunoglobulin gene superfamily, there are antigenic
relationships in the carbohydrate moieties of MAG and
glycoproteins of the immune system. Interestingly, the
HNK-1 reactive structure is also found on other neural
members of the family such as N-CAM, and the possible
significance of this is discussed in more detail below.

In rat brain, MAG occurs in two forms with identical
extracellular domains but differing in the length of the
C-terminal cytoplasmic tails (Lai et al, 1987; Salzer et
al, 1987; Tropak et al, 1988). The two forms are
generated by alternative splicing of the mRNA, thus
showing another similarity to N-CAM which occurs in
several forms with differing C-terminal domains due to
alternative splicing (Edelman, 1986). The two forms of
MAG are developmentally regulated in the CNS; the longer
MAG molecule is the principal form early in development
during the active phase of myelination and the shorter
molecule gradually becomes the principal form with
maturation. In the PNS, MAG appears to occur primarily as
the shorter form at all stages of development (Frail et
al, 1985; Noronha et al, 1988; Tropak et al, 1988).

An interesting property of the cytoplasmic domains is the presence of a number of potential phosphorylation sites for calcium-calmodulin dependent kinase, protein kinase C and tyrosine kinase (Arquint et al, 1987; Lai et al, 1987, Lai et al, 1987). Experimental data showing the phosphorylation of CNS MAG *in vivo* and *in vitro* have recently been reported (Edwards et al, 1988; Edwards et al, 1989).

FUNCTION OF P0 AND MAG IN THE GENERATION OF PNS MYELIN SHEATHS.

P0 and MAG play important, but very different, roles in the formation and maintenance of PNS myelin sheaths. As described in more detail below, the generation of compact PNS myelin may involve the removal of MAG from membranes that are dynamically expanding to create the spiraled structure and its replacement with the smaller P0 protein of tightly layered myelin. The extracellular surfaces of Schwann cell membranes in compact PNS myelin are separated by a very small distance estimated to be about 2 nm in electron micrographs (Trapp and Quarles, 1982), and as mentioned earlier it is believed that the tight apposition of these membranes may be stabilized by homophilic binding of the immunoglobulin domains of P0 molecules on one layer to those on the adjacent layer (Fig. 3). On the other hand, membranes containing the larger MAG molecule with 5 Ig-like domains are always separated by a larger 12-14 nm space (Trapp and Quarles, 1982), and it was postulated that MAG functions to stabilize the greater spacing of these membranes. One example of this larger distance is the periaxonal space between the inner Schwann cell membrane and the axolemma (Fig. 4A). Strong correlative evidence suggesting MAG is functionally involved in maintaining this space was obtained by immunocytochemical studies (Trapp et al, 1984) of a pathological situation in quaking mice in which this space broke down in the absence of MAG (Fig. 4B). MAG is also present in other incompletely compacted regions of PNS myelin sheaths such as Schmidt-Lanterman incisures, lateral loops and the outer mesaxon where extracellular surfaces of adjacent Schwann cell membranes are similarly separated by 12-14 nm. Therefore it was hypothesized that

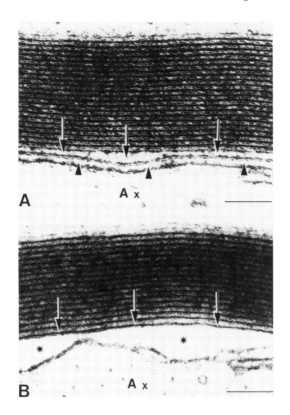

Figure 4. Electron micrographs of myelinated fibers in L4 ventral root of an 11-month old quaking mouse. A. Normally myelinated fiber in which a 12-14 nm periaxonal space (arrow heads) separates the inner Schwann cell membrane containing MAG from the extracellular leaflet of the axolemma. A Schwann cell cytoplasmic collar (arrows) separates the cytoplasmic leaflet of the inner myelin lamella from the cytoplasmic leaflet of the periaxonal Schwann cell membrane. B. Abnormal fiber in which MAG is missing from the periaxonal Schwann cell membrane and there is a dilation of the periaxonal space (asterisks). Also, in the absence of MAG, the cytoplasmic leaflet of the periaxonal membrane fuses with the cytoplasmic leaflet of the inner compact myelin lamella to form an additional major dense line (arrows). Ax, axon. Bars are 0.1 μm. Reproduced from Trapp et al, 1984 with permission.

MAG could also be involved in maintaining the spacing of
these apposed Schwann cell membranes(Trapp and Quarles,
1982; Trapp et al, 1984), and it is possible that this
could occur by homophilic binding of MAG on one membrane
to MAG on the adjacent membrane. However, since MAG is
not expressed on axonal membranes its role in maintaining
the periaxonal space could involve interaction of MAG of
the inner Schwann cell membrane with another member of the
Ig superfamily that is on the axolemmal surface. The
locations of MAG in various Schwann cell membranes
described above were originally demonstrated by comparison
of immunostained 1μm epon sections with adjacent thin
sections examined by conventional electron microscopy
(Trapp and Quarles, 1982), but these locations have more
recently been confirmed by direct electron microscopic
immunocytochemistry using colloidal gold-labelled second
antibodies (Martini and Schachner, 1986; Trapp et al,
1989a).

In addition to the 12-14 nm spacing of extracellular
surfaces of MAG-containing Schwann cell membranes, there
is always cytoplasm present at the inner surface of these
membranes (Trapp and Quarles, 1982). Furthermore, in the
pathological situation occurring in quaking mutants shown
in Fig. 4B, the cytoplasmic, periaxonal Schwann cell
collar is lost in the absence of MAG. Therefore, it was
postulated that in addition to maintaining the spacing of
extracellular membrane surfaces, MAG could help to
maintain intracellular cytoplasmic pockets, possibly by
interacting with cytoskeletal elements (Trapp et al,
1984).

The structural function of MAG in maintaining
membrane periodicity proposed above is expressed in static
terms. However, as a membrane-spanning molecule
interacting with the cytoskeleton at one end and with the
surfaces of adjacent cell membranes at the other, it could
play a very dynamic role in the generation of spiralled
myelin sheaths. Although myelin membrane expansion may
occur at many sites simultaneously, ultimately generation
of the spiralled structure is thought to involve movement
of the inner tongue process around the axon. MAG has been
shown to co-localize with F-actin and other cytoskeletal
elements in myelinating Schwann cells (Fig. 5) (Trapp et
al, 1989a). MAG in the membranes of the inner tongue
process could function to transmit chemo-mechanical forces

involved in generating the spiral by interacting with
cytoskeletal elements such as actin at one end as well as
with adjacent membrane surfaces at the other. This is
illustrated schematically in Figure 6. MAG could bind to
another member of the immunoglobulin superfamily on the
axolemma, and to another member or to itself on the
adjacent Schwann cell membrane. Schmidt-Lanterman
incisures are other structures in PNS myelin sheaths where
MAG could be involved in a dynamic process of membrane
modeling. In these locations, MAG could similarly
interact with cytoskeletal elements and adjacent membrane
surfaces (possibly by homophilic binding) to transmit
chemo-mechanical forces involved in the redistribution of
the cytoplasmic pockets in the sheath.

The remyelinating ventral roots of aging quaking
mice have provided a useful system in which to investigate
the role of P0 and MAG in myelinogenesis since they have a
defect in the conversion of loosely layered mesaxon
membranes to compact myelin (Trapp, 1988). Immunocytochemical investigation of this system has indicated that
the conversion of loosely spiraled, MAG-containing,
mesaxon membranes to compact PNS myelin involves the
removal of MAG and the insertion of P0. Figure 7 shows a
mesaxon membrane encircling an axon 5 times with abundant
cytoplasm between the layers. This mesaxon contains MAG
but no P0. However, intermediate stages exist in which
MAG and P0 are both present in the mesaxon membrane. For
example, Figure 8 shows a fiber where a loosely layered
mesaxon encircles the axon 10 times with little or no
compaction. These membranes are very rich in MAG and
contain small and variable amounts of P0. Figure 9 shows
a sheath which contains many uncompacted membranes on the
left that are rich in both P0 and MAG as well as compacted
membranes on the right that contain P0 but no MAG. In
membranes containing both P0 and MAG, the periodicity is
dictated by the larger MAG molecule so they have the
characteristic 12-14 nm spacing of the extracellular
surfaces and sparse cytoplasm at the inner surface. In
order to convert these membranes containing both
glycoproteins to compact myelin it is necessary to remove
the MAG so that homophilic binding of smaller P0 molecules
can occur and stabilize the intraperiod line and to allow
the cytoplasmic sides to converge to form the major dense
line. In areas of developing sheaths that contain both P0
and MAG, it is feasible that P0 interacts with MAG

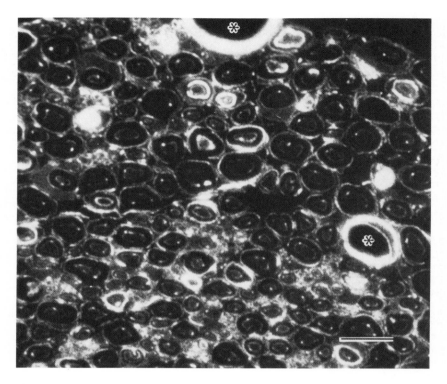

Figure 5 - Cytochemical localization of F-actin in a 1 μm
cryosection of 7-day-old rat sciatic nerve demonstrated by
rhodamine-labelled phallicidin binding.   F-actin was
detected in myelinated fibers, unmyelinated fibers and
around blood vessels (asterisks).   All myelinated fibers
contained a periaxonal ring of F-actin staining that
included an intense dot corresponding to the inner tongue
process.   Further cytochemical results at the light and
electron microscopic level (Trapp et al, 1989a) showed the
colocalization of F-actin, spectrin and MAG in periaxonal
membranes, Schmidt-Lanterman incisures, paranodal loops
and inner and outer mesaxons of myelinating Schwann cells.
The findings indicate that plasma membrane linkage of F-
actin in Schwann cells is likely to occur via spectrin and
raise the possibility that microfilaments interact with
the cytoplasmic domains of MAG. Scale bar: 10 μm.
Reproduced from Trapp et al (1989a) with permission.

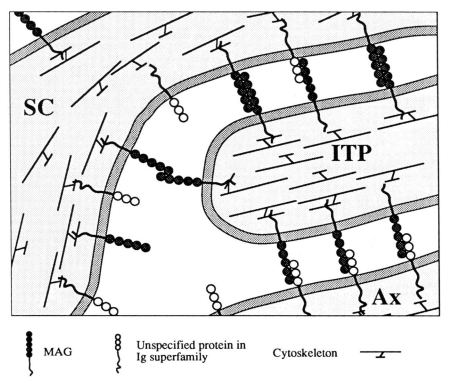

MAG

Unspecified protein in
Ig superfamily

Cytoskeleton

SC: Schwann cell   ITP: inner tongue process   Ax: axon

Figure 6. Diagrammatic representation of how MAG may
function to transmit chemo-mechanical forces involved in
the movement of the inner tongue process (ITP) of the
Schwann cell around the axon to form the spiralled mesaxon.
The extracellular domains of MAG molecules in the ITP may
interact with Ig-like domains of other unspecified members
of the Ig superfamily on the axolemma and with those of
other members of the family or itself on the adjacent
Schwann cell membrane. The cytoplasmic domains of MAG may
bind to cytoskeletal elements of the Schwann cell. Thus,
MAG could transmit chemo-mechanical forces between
contractile elements of the cytoskeleton and adjacent
membrane surfaces during generation of the spiralled
mesaxon.

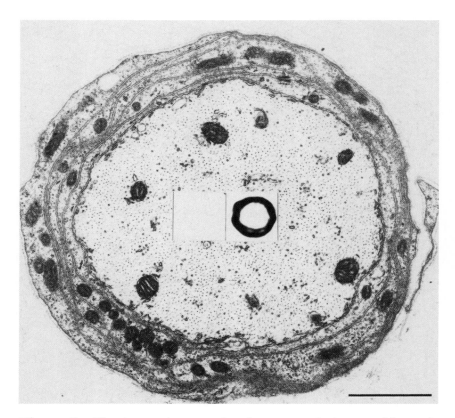

Figure 7. Electron micrograph of an axon being myelinated
in the ventral root of an 11-month old quaking mouse with
serial, adjacent semi-thin sections immunostained for P0
(left inset) and MAG (right inset). The mesaxon process
encircles the axon 5 times and contains abundant
cytoplasm. It was stained intensely for MAG, but P0 was
not detectable. Bar, 1μm. Reproduced from Trapp (1988)
with permission.

molecules that are laterally adjacent to it in the same
layer of the spiral or with MAG molecules across from it
in the next layer of the spiral. Such interactions between
the two proteins could play a role in controlling the
compaction process. The transition from MAG-containing

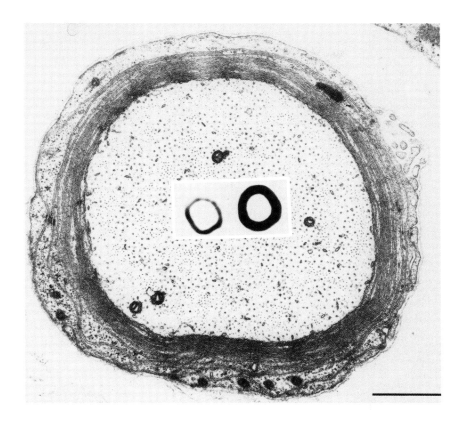

Figure 8. Electron micrograph of an axon being myelinated
in the ventral root of an 11-month old quaking mouse with
serial, adjacent semi-thin sections immunostained for P0
(left inset) and MAG (right inset). The mesaxon process
encircles the axon 10 times and contains sparse cytoplasm
and detectable levels of both P0 and MAG. Compared to MAG
staining, the ring of P0 staining was thinner and varied
in intensity. Bar, 1μm. Reproduced from Trapp (1988) with
permission.

mesaxon membranes to P0-containing compact myelin is
illustrated schematically in Figure 10. The studies of
Trapp (1988) suggesting this molecular mechanism of
myelination also suggest that the failure of mesaxons in

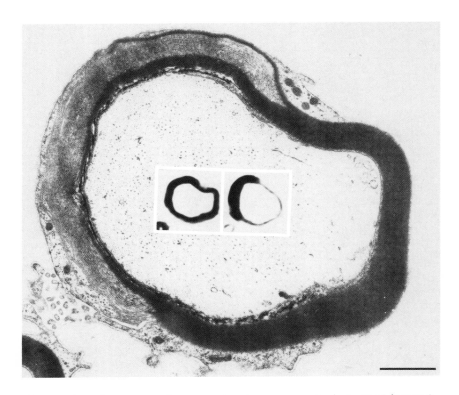

Figure 9. Electron micrograph of an axon being myelinated
in the ventral root of an 11-month old quaking mouse with
serial, adjacent semi-thin sections immunostained for P0
(left inset) and MAG (right inset). The axon is partially
surrounded by noncompact Schwann cell membranes (left
half) that are continuous with compact myelin lamellae
(right half). The intensity and thickness of P0 staining
were similar over the noncompact and compact membranes.
The noncompact Schwann cell membranes on the left were
stained intensely for MAG, but MAG staining was restricted
to the inner periaxonal Schwann cell membrane on the
right. Bar, 1μm. Reproduced from Trapp (1988) with
permission.

quaking mice to convert to compact myelin is due to a
deficiency in the ability to remove MAG. The mechanism by

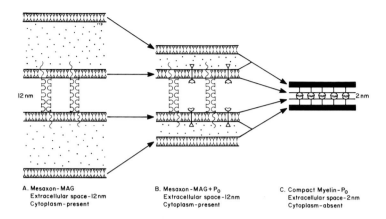

A. Mesaxon-MAG
Extracellular space-12nm
Cytoplasm-present

B. Mesaxon-MAG+P₀
Extracellular space-12nm
Cytoplasm-present

C. Compact Myelin-P₀
Extracellular space-2nm
Cytoplasm-absent

Figure 10. Hypothesis about the distribution, orientation
and function of P0 and MAG during conversion of mesaxon
membranes to compact myelin. P0 and MAG are shown only in
the inner two membrane bilayers. During the initial
wrapping of the mesaxon the membranes contain MAG but
little or no P0 (A). The bulky extracellular domains of
MAG maintain a constant 12-14 nm spacing between
extracellular surfaces possibly by homophilic binding
between the Ig-like domains of apposing MAG molecules. As
the mesaxon spiral is lengthened, P0 protein is inserted
(B). However, the spacing between extracellular surfaces
is still controlled by the larger MAG molecules. The
cytoplasmic domains of MAG interact with cytoskeleton and
prevent the fusion of cytoplasmic leaflets of these P0-
containing membranes. When the concentration of P0 in the
membranes becomes high enough, MAG is removed from the
spiralled mesaxon and compact myelin is formed (C). The
spacing of the extracellular surfaces in the compact
myelin is controlled by homotypic interactions of the Ig-
like domains of P0 molecules as suggested by Lemke et al
(1988). The close packing of the cytoplasmic leaflets in
compact myelin may be mediated in part by homophilic
interactions of the cytoplasmic domains of P0 or the
interaction of these domains with acidic lipids in the
bilayer (also see Figure 3). Reproduced from Trapp (1988)
with permission.

which MAG is removed in normal myelination and whether the biochemical abnormalities of MAG in quaking mice described below are related to the deficiency in its removal remain to be determined.

FUNCTION OF MAG IN CNS MYELINATION.

The periaxonal localization of MAG in developing and mature myelin sheaths in the CNS (Sternberger et al, 1979) suggests that it is involved in oligodendrocyte-axon interactions. In fact, this may be its principal function in the formation and maintenance of CNS myelin sheaths, since it does not appear to be present in paranodal regions, incisures or the outer mesaxon in a manner analogous to the PNS (Trapp, Andrews, Cootauco and Quarles in preparation). Since oligodendrocytes send out multiple processes and form many internodes of myelin, the primary site of growth of the spiral is thought to be at the inner tongue process adjacent to the axon. Although spiraling of loose mesaxon membranes is not as prominent in the CNS as the PNS, MAG may nevertheless play a role in transmitting chemo-mechanical forces involved in generating the spiral much as was hypothesized above for the PNS. Also, MAG must similarly be removed from oligodendrocyte membranes before compact myelin is formed. However, in the CNS it is not replaced by another member of the family, since proteolipid protein (which is not in the family) appears to be involved in stabilizing the intraperiod line of compact CNS myelin (Fig. 3).

An interesting difference with regard to immunocytochemical staining of MAG in the PNS and CNS is that MAG is generally not detectable by light microscope immunocytochemistry in the cytoplasm of actively myelinating Schwann cells whereas myelinating oligodendrocyte cytoplasm is heavily stained for MAG (Sternberger et al, 1979; Trapp and Quarles, 1982). The absence of staining in Schwann cell perinuclear regions must mean that MAG is efficiently transported to the myelin spiral and does not accumulate to detectable levels in the rough endoplasmic reticulum and Golgi apparatus. By contrast there is strong staining for MAG in oligodendrocytes of developing brain, and much of the staining appears particulate (Sternberger et al, 1979). Recent electron microscopic immunocytochemistry indicates that oligodendrocytes and their processes contain MAG-rich, multi-vesicular bodies (MVBs) (Trapp et al, 1989b). The MVBs are also found in the outer tongue processes and in paranodal or periaxonal cytoplasm. In addition to these MAG-enriched MVBs, a less intense, diffuse staining of oligodendrocyte cytoplasm is also present and probably represents MAG in small vesicles. The findings suggest that translocation of MAG between oligodendrocyte cell bodies and myelin internodes occurs in part via MVBs. The bodies may be moving in an anterograde or retrograde direction, or both, and may also carry other molecules important to the process of myelination.

PROPERTIES OF MAG RELEVANT TO ITS FUNCTION IN MYELINATION.

Many of the properties of MAG deduced from the sequencing of cDNAs are compatible with a function for MAG in cell-cell or membrane-membrane interactions and suggest ways that such interactions could be modulated. The propensity of proteins with Ig-like domains to bind to themselves or other members of the family has already been discussed. In addition, MAG has an Arg-Gly-Asp sequence in domain 1 (Arquint et al, 1987; Lai et al, 1987; Salzer et al, 1987) suggesting that some aspects of its interactions with other cells could involve a receptor in the integrin class (Rusolahti and Pierschbacher, 1986). The oligosaccharides of MAG could also be involved in or modulate interactions of the extracellular domains. Since the HNK-1/L2 carbohydrate epitope which is expressed on MAG has been found primarily on cell adhesion proteins, it was proposed that it could play a functional role in such interactions and some evidence to support this was reported (Kruse et al, 1984; 1985; Keilhauer et al, 1985). The two developmentally regulated forms of MAG with different C-terminal cytoplasmic domains could bind to the cytoskeleton in different ways. Interactions with cytoskeleton could also be modulated by phosphorylation of this part of the molecule. These chemical properties plus the correlative immunocytochemical investigations summarized in the previous section provide compelling circumstantial evidence suggesting that MAG is involved in membrane-membrane interactions and also binds to cytoskeletal elements. However, direct evidence indicating that MAG plays a role in the postulated functions is limited at this time.

Experiments on the effects of an anti-MAG monoclonal antibody on neural cell interactions have been interpreted to indicate that MAG does possess adhesive properties that would enable it to mediate such interactions (Polterak et al, 1987). Using monolayer cultures as target cells and single cell suspensions as probe cells, it was demonstrated that Fab fragments of the monoclonal anti-MAG antibody inhibited oligodendrocyte to neuron and oligodendrocyte to oligodendrocyte adhesion, but not oligodendrocyte to astrocyte adhesion. One difficulty in the interpretation of these experiments is that the interactions studied were those between oligodendrocytes and small cerebellar neurons (or between oligodendrocytes) and not between oligodendrocytes and axons of large neurons that would be myelinated under physiological circumstances. The physiological relevance is also not clear because *in vivo* MAG is not detectable on the plasma membranes of oligodendrocyte perikarya (Trapp, unpublished results). Another factor that may be relevant to these experiments on cell-cell interactions is that MAG that has been denatured by exposure to lithium diiodosalicylate (LIS) or SDS during isolation (Quarles et al, 1983) may have different properties and give rise to a different population of antibodies than native MAG. Indications that this may be the case is discussed to some extent by Polterak et al (1987), but much more work is needed to substantiate the postulated role of MAG in physiologically relevant, cell-cell interactions during myelinogenesis.

A more direct demonstration that MAG is at least capable of binding to normal target axons for myelination was achieved by demonstrating that MAG-containing liposomes bound to neurites in dorsal root ganglia and spinal cord cultures, and the binding was inhibited by the monoclonal antibody described above (Polterak et al, 1987). Again the importance of the physical state of the MAG was indicated by the fact that this experiment was done with MAG isolated from non-ionic detergent lysates, whereas MAG isolated by the LIS-phenol method could not be incorporated into liposomes. Another indication of the adhesive propeties of MAG comes from the recent report that neurites of retinal explants grow better over cultures of heterologous (non-glial) cells that have been transfected with MAG than of control cells (Salzer et al, 1989).

The binding of MAG to extracellular matrix constituents has also been investigated (Fahrig et al, 1987). These experiments revealed high affinity binding of MAG to heparin and several types of collagen, but not to laminin, fibronectin, N-CAM, L1 or itself. These experiments were done with MAG isolated from mouse brain with neutral detergent as well as with a soluble, slightly smaller form of MAG. The soluble smaller MAG may arise by proteolysis of intact MAG and correspond to dMAG (Sato et al, 1982; 1984; Fahrig et al, 1987). N-CAM has also been shown to have a heparin binding domain which appears to function both in cell-cell and cell-substratum interactions (Cole and Glazer, 1986). The physiological significance of the binding of MAG to heparin and collagen is not known at this time, but suggests that MAG could play a role in the interaction of cells with extracellular matrix. Immunocytochemical observations at the electron microscope level were interpreted to indicate that, in addition to its location in Schwann cell membranes, MAG may be present in the extracellular matrix of peripheral nerve (Martini and Schachner, 1986). Although all forms of MAG so far identified have a trans-membrane domain, it is possible that a secreted form of MAG similar to that recently reported for N-CAM (Gower et al, 1988) will be found

The failure to observe binding of MAG to itself or to N-CAM or L1 (Fahrig et al, 1987) argues against homophilic binding or heterophilic binding to these well known Ig superfamily members as an aspect of MAG function. It should be kept in mind, however, that these negative findings apply only to the conditions of the experiments and do not necessarily rule out these types of interactions under appropriate conditions. With regard to homophilic binding, the negative experiments were done with CNS MAG, and the only known location where MAG could bind to itself is in adjacent Schwann cell membranes of the PNS. The binding properties of MAG that have been studied so far are intriguing, but must be considered preliminary at this time. Much more information is needed before a comprehensive understanding of MAG function in myelin formation and maintenance can be achieved.

Some clues about the normal molecular mechanisms of MAG function may be obtained from investigation of situations in which MAG is abnormal. As described above, some morphological abnormalities in quaking mice appear to be related to the fact that MAG is not present in parts of the periaxonal Schwann cell membrane and is not adequately removed from the spiraled mesaxon to permit myelin compaction (Trapp et al, 1984; Trapp, 1988). Biochemical abnormalities in the structure and metabolism of MAG have also been found in quaking mice and may be responsible in part for the pathology. The biochemical abnormalities are not caused by a primary mutation of the MAG gene, since the quaking mutation is on chromosome 17 (Hogan and Greenfield, 1984) whereas the MAG gene is on chromosome 7 (Barton et al, 1987; D'Eustachio et al, 1988). However, it may be that the quaking mutation directly affects the synthesis and/or posttranslational processing of MAG. *In vitro* translation experiments (Frail and Braun, 1985) and Western blotting with antibodies that distinguish between the two forms of MAG (Noronha et al, 1988) have shown that Quaking mice have primarily the shorter form and little or none of the longer form. Paradoxically, most of the completely processed MAG molecules made in both the CNS and PNS of quaking mice are slightly larger than those of controls (Fig. 11) (Matthieu et al, 1974; Inuzuka et al, 1987). This suggests that MAG in quaking mice may be more extensively glycosylated than that in controls. Preliminary results in our laboratory indicate that MAG in quaking mice contains more sialic acid and less of the HNK-1/L2 carbohydrate epitope than that in control mice (Noronha and Quarles, unpublished results). Abnormal processing of MAG oligosaccharides in quaking mice was also indicated by an increased incorporation of radioactive mannose relative to fucose (Konat et al, 1987). The minor, lower molecular weight band seen exclusively in the quaking samples in Figure 11 may indicate the presence of a small amount of MAG with high mannose oligosaccharides in the mutant. The manner in which the altered polypeptide and carbohydrate moieties of MAG in the quaking mutant may affect the function of this glycoprotein remains to be established.

FUNCTION OF N-CAM AND L1 IN MYELINATION.

P0 and MAG are members of the immunoglobulin superfamily that have their primary function in

1 2 3

Figure 11. Western blot of brainstem homogenates from control (lane 1) and quaking (lanes 2 and 3) 36-day-old mice immunostained for MAG. The higher apparent molecular weight for most of the MAG from quaking mice is apparent. In addition, the quaking samples had a very minor, smaller stained band of unknown significance. Total homogenate protein electrophoresed: control, 20 μg; quaking, 60 and 120 μg in lanes 2 and 3, respectively. Reproduced from Inuzuka et al (1987) with permission.

myelination. However, myelin forming cells express N-CAM and/or L1 and these adhesion proteins may also play a role in myelination, especially in the very early stages. Martini and Schachner (1986) have shown that Schwann cells are N-CAM and L1 positive when they first contact each other, and MAG is not detected until the early stages of mesaxon spiraling. At this stage, L1 ceases to be detectable and N-CAM is greatly reduced. Therefore, it may be that N-CAM or L1 are involved in the initial interaction of Schwann cells and axons and that MAG takes over this interaction as the myelination proceeds. These authors report a similar sequence of events during remyelination (Martini and Schachner, 1988), but Trapp et al (1984) observed that MAG was present at the time of first Schwann cell-axon interactions during remyelination. Also, biochemical studies showed that during normal development of peripheral nerve, MAG accumulates well before P0 (Willison et al, 1987). As described above, MAG appears to be involved in generation of the mesaxon spiral and is replaced by P0 during compaction. Thus, PNS myelination involves sequential functioning of members of immunoglobulin gene superfamily.

N-CAM occurs in 180, 140 and 120 kD forms with different C-termini due to alternative splicing of the mRNA (Edelman, 1986), and the smallest form is linked to membranes by a phosphatidyl inositol linkage (Barthels et al, 1987; He et al, 1986; Hemperly et al 1986). Oligodendrocytes express N-CAM, and interestingly it appears to be exclusively the 120 kD form (Bhat and Silberburg, 1986; 1988). Based on developmental studies and other observations, Bhat and Silberburg (1988) hypothesized that N-CAM-120 on oligodendrocytes must come in contact with N-CAM-180 of axons during myelination.

CONCLUSIONS AND PERSPECTIVES.

In summary, it appears that myelination involves some members of the Ig gene superfamily that function primarily or exclusively in the context of myelination (P0 and MAG) and others that perform more general roles in neuron-neuron, neuron-glia, and glia-glia interactions in the nervous system (e.g. N-CAM and L1). Also, since myelin and myelin-forming cells contain a heterogeneous population of glycoproteins many of which are not yet well characterized (Quarles, 1979 and in press), additional members of the Ig superfamily that play a role in myelination are likely to be identified. Members of the family probably function both cooperatively and sequentially during the cell-cell and membrane-membrane interactions occurring during myelination.

At this point, our understanding of the precise molecular mechanisms by which these glycoproteins function during myelination is at a very early stage. However, the recent determination from cDNAs of complete amino acid sequences for many of the proteins and the application of techniques of molecular biology should result in the rapid acceleration of the field. A principal subject to be addressed will be the capacity of members of the family to exhibit homophilic binding and to bind with other specified members of the family under physiological circumstances. Once binding has been established it will be necessary to establish which domains of the molecules are involved in the interactions. This research will probably involve inhibition of interactions with specific antibodies, oligosaccharides and synthetic peptides as well as transfection of cells with the genes for these proteins and site-directed mutagenesis. It is likely that a heavy reliance on model systems for studying the interactions will be required, since many of the *in situ* glial-axonal and membrane-membrane interactions during myelinogenesis occur at sequestered locations which are not readily accessible to perturbation by external agents. In addition to extracellular interactions, investigation of the interaction of these transmembrane proteins with cytoskeletal elements will probably be central to a molecular understanding of the dynamic aspects of myelination. Finally, in addition to the nature of the molecular interactions, it is important to determine factors controlling the expression and post-translational processing of proteins in the immunoglobulin superfamily by myelin-forming cells and axons.

REFERENCES

Abo T, Balch CM (1981). A differentiation antigen of human NK and K cells identified by a monoclonal antibody (HNK-1). J Immunol 127: 1024- 1029.
Arquint M, Roder J, Chia L, Down J, Wilkerson D, Bayley H,

Braun P, Dunn R (1987). Molecular cloning and the
primary structure of the myelin-associated glycoprotein.
Proc Natl Acad Sci (USA) 84: 600-604.

Barthels D, Santoni M-J, Wille W , Rupper C, Chaiz J-C,
Hirsch M-R, Fontcilla-Camps J-C, Goridis C (1987).
Isolation and nucleotide sequence of mouse N-CAM cDNA
that codes for a Mr 79,000 polypeptide without a
membrane spanning region. EMBO J 6:907-914.

Barton DE, Arquint M, Roder J, Dunn R, Franke U (1987).
The myelin-associated glycoprotein gene: mapping to
human chromosome 19 and mouse chromosome 7 and
expression in quivering mice. Genomics 1: 107-112.

Bhat S, Silberburg DH (1986). Oligodendrocyte cell
adhesion molecules are related to neural cell adhesion
molecule (N-CAM). J Neurosci 6: 3384-3354.

Bhat S, Silberburg DH (1988). Developmental expression of
neural cell adhesion molecules of oligodendrocytes in
vivo and in culture. J. Neurochem. 50: 1830-1838.

Cole GJ, Glaser L (1986). A heparin binding domain from
N-CAM is involved in neural cell substratum adhesion J.
Cell Biol. 102: 403-412.

Cunningham BA, Hemperly JJ, Murray BA, Prediger EA,
Brackenberry R, Edelman GM (1987) Neural adhesion
molecule: Structure, immunoglobulin-like domains, cell
surface modulation and alternative RNA splicing. Science
236:799-806.

D'Eustachio P, Colman DR, Salzer JL (1988). Chromosomal
location of the mouse gene that encodes the myelin-
associated glycoproteins. J Neurochem 50:589-593.

Edelman GM (1986). Cell adhesion molecules in the
regulation of animal form and tissue pattern. Ann Rev
Cell Biol 259: 14857 - 14862.

Edelman GM (1987). CAMs and Igs: Cell adhesion and the
evolutionary origins of immunity. Immunological Reviews
100: 11-45.

Edwards AM, Arquint M, Braun PE, Roder JC, Dunn RJ, Dawson
T, Bell JC (1988). Myelin-associated glycoprotein: a
cell adhesion molecule of oligodendrocytes is
phosphorylated in brain. Mol. Cell Biol. 8: 2655-2658.

Edwards AM, Braun P, Bell JC (1989). Phosphorylation of
myelin-àssociated glycoprotein in vivo and in vitro
occurs only in the cytoplasmic domain of the large
isoform. J Neurochem 52: 317-320.

Fahrig T, Landa C, Pesheva P, Kuhn K, Schachner M (1987).
Characterization of binding properties of the myelin-
associated glycoprotein to extracellular matrix

constituents. EMBO J 6: 2875-2873.

Frail DE, Braun PE (1985). Abnormal expression of the myelin-associated glycoprotein in the central nervous system of dysmyelinating mutant mice. J Neurochem 45: 1071-1075.

Frail DE, Webster H. deF, Braun PE (1985). Developmental expression of the myelin-associated glycoprotein in the peripheral nervous system is different from that in the central nervous system. J Neurochem 45: 1308-1310.

Gay D, Maddion P, Sekaly R, Talle MA, Godfrey M, Long E, Goldstein G, Chess L, Axel R, Kappler J, Merrack P (1987). Functional interaction between human T-cell protein CD4 and the major histocompatibility complex HLA-DR antigen. Nature 328: 626-629.

Gower HJ, Barton H, Elsom VL, Thompson J, Moore SE, Dickson G, Walsh FS (1988). Alternative slicing generates a secreted form of N-CAM in muscle and brain. Cell 55: 955-964.

Harrelson AL, Goodman CS (1988). Growth cone guidance in insects: Fasciclin II is a member of the immunoglobulin superfamily. Science 242: 700-708.

He HT, Finne J, Goridis C (1987). Phosphatidyl inositol is involved in the membrane attachment of N-CAM, the smallest component of the neural cell adhesion molecule. EMBO J 5: 2489-2500.

Hemperly JJ, Edelman GM, Cunningham BA (1986). cDNA clones of the neural cell adhesion molecule (N-CAM) lacking a membrane-spanning region consistent with evidence for membrane attachment via a phosphatidylinositol intermediate. Proc Natl Acad Sci USA 83: 9822-9826.

Hogan EL, Greenfield S (1984). Animal models of genetic disorders of myelin. In Morell P (ed).: "Myelin," New York: Plenum Press, pp. 489-534.

Inuzuka T, Johnson D, Quarles RH (1987). Myelin-associated glycoprotein in the central and peripheral nervous system of quaking mice. J Neurochem 49: 597-602.

Keilhauer G, Faissner A, Schachner M (1985). Differential inhibition of neurone-neurone, neurone-astrocyte and astrocyte-astrocyte adhesion by L1, L2 and N-CAM antibodies. Nature 316: 728-730.

Konat G, Hogan EL, Leskawa KC, Gantt G, Singh I (1987). Abnormal glycosylation of myelin-associated glycoprotein in quaking mouse brain. Neurochem Int 10: 555-558.

Kruse J, Mailhammer R, Wernecke A, Faissner I, Sommer C, Goridis C, Schachner M (1984). Neural cell adhesion molecules and myelin-associated glycoprotein share a common carbohydrate moiety recognized by monoclonal antibodies L2 and HNK-1. Nature 311: 153-155.

Kruse J, Keilhauer G, Faissner A, Sommer C, Goridis C, Schachner M (1985). The J1 glycoprotein - a novel nervous system adhesion molecule of the L2?HNK-1 family. Nature 316: 728-730.

Lai C, Brow MA, Nave KA, Noronha AB, Quarles RH, Bloom FE, Milner RJ, Sutcliffe JG (1987). Two forms of 1B236/myelin-associated glycoprotein, a cell adhesion molecule for postnatal neural development, are produced by alternative splicing. Proc Natl Acad Sci USA 84: 4337-4341.

Lai C, Watson JB, Bloom FE, Sutcliffe JG, Milner RJ (1988). Neural protein 1B236/MAG defines a subgroup of the immunoglobulin superfamily. Immunological Rev 100: 129-149.

Lemke G, Axel R (1985). Isolation and sequence of a cDNA encoding the major structural protein of peripheral myelin. Cell 40: 501-508.

Lemke G, Lamar E, Patterson J (1988). Isolation and analysis of the gene encoding peripheral myelin protein zero. Neuron 1: 73-83.

Martini R, Schachner M (1986). Immunoelectron microscopic localization of neural cell adhension molecules (L1, N-CAM, and MAG) and their shared carbohydrate epitope and myelin basic protein in developing sciatic nerve. J Cell Biol 103: 2439-2448.

Martini R, Schachner M (1988). Immunoelectron microscopic localization of neural cell adhension molecules (L1, N-CAM, and myelin-associated glycoprotein) in regenerating adult mouse sciatic nerve. J Cell Biol 106: 1735-1746.

Matthieu J-M, Brady RO, Quarles RH (1974). Anomalies of myelin-associated glycoprotein in Quaking mice. J Neurochem 22: 291-296.

Matthieu J-M, Quarles RH, Poduslo J, Brady RO (1975). ^{35}S-Sulfate incorporation into myelin glycoproteins: I Central nervous system Biochim Biophys Acta 392: 159-166.

Moos M, Tacke R, Scherer H, Teplow D, Fruh K, Schachner M (1988). Neural adhesion molecule L1 as a member of the immunoglobulin superfamily with binding domains similar to fibronectin. Nature 334:701-703.

Morell P, Quarles RH, Norton WT (1989) Formation, structure and biochemistry of myelin. In Siegel GJ, Agranoff BW, Albers RW, Molinoff PB (eds): "Basic

Neurochemistry," New York: Raven Press, pp109-136.

Mostov KE, Friedlander M, Blobel G (1984). The receptor for trans-epithelial transport of IgA and IgM contains multiple immunoglobulin domains. Nature 308: 37-43.

Murray N, Steck AJ (1984). Indication of a possible role in a demyelinating neuropathy for an antigen shared between myelin and NK cells. Lancet 1: 711-713.

Noronha AB, Ilyas AA, Antonicek H, Schachner M, Quarles RH (1986). Molecular specificity of L2 monoclonal antibodies that bind to carbohydrate determinants of neural cell adhesion molecules their resemblance to other monoclonal antibodies recognizing the myelin-associated glycoprotein. Brain Research 385: 237-244.

Noronha A, Hammer J, Milner R, Sutcliffe G Quarles R (1988). Immunological characterization of MAG in normal and mutant CNS and PNS Trans Amer Soc Neurochem 19: 118.

Noronha AB, Baba H, Moller J, Inuzuka T, Hammer JA, Agrawal H, Quarles RH (1989). Post-translational processing of the myelin-associated glycoprotein. J Neurochem 51S: in press.

Noronha AB, Hammer JA, Lai E, Kiel M, Milner RJ, Sutcliffe JG, Quarles RH (1989). The myelin-associated glycoprotein (MAG) and the rat brain-specific 1B236 protein: Mapping of epitopes and demonstration of immunological identity. J Mol Neurosci: in press.

O'Shannessy DJ, Willison HJ, Inuzuka T, Dobersen MJ, Quarles RH (1985). The species distribution of nervous system antigens that react with anti-myelin-associated glycoprotein antibodies. J Neuroimmunol 9: 255-268.

Poltorak M, Sadoul R, Keilhauer G, Landa C, Fahrig T, Schachner M (1987). Myelin-associated glycoprotein, a member of the L2/HNK-1 family of neural cell adhesion molecules, is involved in neuron-oligodendrocyte and oligodendrocyte-oligodendrocyte interaction. J Cell Biol 105: 1893-1899.

Quarles RH (1979). Glycoproteins in myelin and myelin-related membranes.In Margolis RU, Margolis RK (eds): "Complex Carbohydrates of Nervous Tissue," New York: Plenum Press, pp 209-233.

Quarles RH (1988). Myelin-associated glycoprotein: Functional and clinical aspects. In Marangos PJ, Campbell IC, Cohen RM (eds) "Neuronal and Glial Proteins: Structure, Function and Clinical Application," San Diego: Academic Press, pp 295-320.

Quarles RH (1989). Glycoproteins of myelin and myelin-forming cells.In Margolis RK, Margolis RU (eds)

"Neurobiology of Glycoconjugates," New York: Plenum Press, in press.

Quarles RH, Barbarash GR, Figlewicz DA McIntyre LJ (1983). Purification and partial characterization of the myelin-associated glycoprotein from adult rat brain. Biochim Biophys Acta 757: 140-143.

Sakamoto Y, Kitamura K, Yoshimura K, Nishijima T, Uyemura K (1987). Complete amino acid sequence of P0 protein in bovine peripheral nerve myelin. J Biol Chem 262: 4208-4214.

Salzer J, Brown M, Pedreza L, Owens G (1989) Use of transfected cells in functional studies of MAG proteins. Trans Amer Soc Neurochem 20: 95

Salzer JL, Holmes WP, Colman DR (1987). The amino acid sequences of the myelin-associated glycoproteins: Homology to the immunoglobulin gene superfamily. J Cell Biol 104: 957-965.

Sato S, Quarles RH, Brady RO (1982). Susceptibility of the myelin-associated glycoprotein and basic protein to a neutral protease in highly purified myelin from human and rat brain. J Neurochem 39: 97-105.

Sato S, Baba H, Tanaka M, Yanagisawa K, Miyatake T (1983). Antigenic determinant shared between myelin-associated glycoprotein from human brain and natural killer cells. Biomed Res 4: 489-493.

Sato S, Yanagisawa K, Miyatake T (1984a). Conversion of myelin-associated glycoprotein (MAG) to a smaller derivative by calcium activated neutral protease (CANP)-like enzyme in myelin and inhibition by E-64 analogue. Neurochem Res 9: 629-635.

Sternberger NH, Quarles RH, Itoyama Y, Webster H deF (1979). Myelin-associated glycoprotein demonstrated immunocytochemically in myelin and myelin forming cells of developing rat. Proc Natl Acad Sci,USA 76, 1510-1514.

Trapp BD (1988). Distribution of the myelin-associated glycoprotein and P0 protein during myelin compaction in quaking mouse peripheral nerve. J Cell Biol 107: 675-685.

Trapp BD, Quarles RH (1982). Presence of myelin-associated glycoprotein correlates with alterations in the periodicity of peripheral myelin. J Cell Biol 92: 877-882.

Trapp BD, Quarles RH, Suzuki K (1984). Immunocytochemical studies of Quaking mice support a role for the myelin-associated glycoprotein in forming and maintaining the periaxonal space and periaxonal cytoplasmic collar in myelinating Schwann cells. J Cell Biol 99: 595-606.

Trapp BD, Griffin JW, Wong M, O'Connell M, Andrews SB (1989a). Co-localization of the myelin-associated glycoprotein and the microfilament components, F-actin and spectrin, in Schwann cells of myelinated nerve fibers. J Neurocytol 18: 47-60..

Trapp BD, Andrews SB, Cootauco C, Quarles RH (1989b). The myelin-associated glycoprotein is enriched in multivesicular bodies during CNS myelination. J Cell Biol 107: 666a.

Tropak MB, Johnson PW, Dunn RJ, Roder JC (1988). Differential splicing of MAG transcripts during CNS and PNS development. Mol Brain Res 4: 143-155.

Uyemura K, Suzuki M, Sakamoto Y, Tanaka S (1987). Structure of P0 protein: Homology to immunoglobulin superfamily. Biomed. Res. 8: 353-357.

Williams AF (1984).The immunoglobulin superfamily takes shape. Nature 308:12-13.

Williams AF (1987). A year in the life of the immuno-globulin superfamily. Immunol Today 8: 298-303.

Williams AF, Gagnon J (1982) Neuronal cell Thy-1 glycoprotein: homology with immunoglobulin. Science 216: 696-703.

Willison HJ, Ilyas AI, O'Shannessy DJ, Pulley M, Trapp BD, Quarles RH (1987). Myelin-associated glycoprotein and related glycoconjugates in developing cat peripheral nerve: a correlative biochemical and morphometric study. J Neurochem 49: 1853-1862.

Dynamic Interactions of Myelin Proteins, pages 81–92

MYELIN BASIC PROTEIN AND MYELINOGENESIS: MORPHOMETRIC
ANALYSIS OF NORMAL, MUTANT AND TRANSGENIC CENTRAL NERVOUS
SYSTEM

H. David Shine, Carol Readhead, Brian Popko,
Leroy Hood and Richard L. Sidman

Center for Biotechnology, Baylor College of
Medicine, Houston, TX 77030 (H.D.S), Division of
Biology, California Institute of Technology,
Pasadena, CA 91125 (C.R., L.H.), Biological
Sciences Research Center, University of North
Carolina School of Medicine, Chapel Hill, NC
27514 (B.P.), Department of Neuropathology,
Harvard Medical School, Boston, MA 02115 (R.L.S.)

INTRODUCTION

Myelinogenesis is a dynamic process requiring highly
interdependent multi-gene expression. Just as in other
developmental systems a perturbation in one gene's
expression will greatly affect the whole myelination process
and may drastically change the end result. An example of
coordinated gene expression in myelinogenesis is
demonstrated when Myelin Basic Protein (MBP) accumulation is
compared to the rate of myelin formation in neonatal rodent
central nervous system (CNS). During the second week after
birth there is a rapid increase in MBP accumulation with a
coincident increase in the rate of myelin formation (Fig.
1). The availability of mouse stocks in which adults express
MBP at levels lower than normal and similar to the net
amounts expressed during the period of myelinogenesis,
provide a means to investigate the link between MBP
expression and myelin formation. These stocks contain
combinations of the shiverer (shi) mutation, the myelin
deficient (shi^{mld}) mutation, an MBP transgene, and the
normal (wild type) MBP gene.

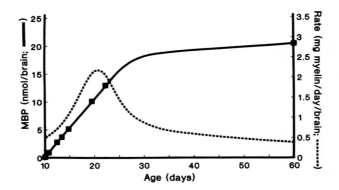

Figure 1. MBP accumulation (Barbarese et al., 1978) and rate of myelination (Norton and Poduslo, 1973). The increase in the rate of myelination in the 10 to 20 days after birth is coincident with rapid accumulation of MBP. Predicted gene doses listed on Table 2 are superimposed on the MBP accumulation curve (■).

Shiverer is an autosomal recessive mutation located on the end away from the centromere of chromosome 18 (Sidman et al., 1985). It arose spontaneously in a colony of Swiss Vancouver mice in 1973 (Biddle et al., 1973). The primary *shi* phenotype is a course action tremor with a frequency of about 12 Hz and varying amplitude that is first detected on about the 12th postnatal day. At roughly 30 days of age *shi* mice begin to have tonic seizures that are elicited by sensory stimuli such as light, sound and cage movement. The frequency and intensity of seizures increases with age and may be responsible for the short life span of *shi* mice (4 to 5 months versus 2 to 3 years in wild type mice). The CNS of a *shi* mouse is virtually devoid of myelin and axons within the CNS are separated by little or no oligodendrocytic membrane, so that often they are touching one another (Fig. 2). Other than the absence of myelin, oligodendrocytes and neurons appear virtually normal. Interestingly, myelin in the peripheral nervous systems (PNS) of these mice displays only subtle abnormalities (Rosenbluth, 1980). MBP is not detected in PNS and CNS tissue in *shi* mice (Dupouey et al., 1979; Kirschner and Ganser, 1980). This, and the fact that the gene for MBP, like the shiverer locus, maps by somatic cell hybridization and *in situ* hybridization to the end of chromosome 18 (Barnett et al., 1985; Roach et al., 1985) suggests that the molecular basis for the *shi* dysmyelinating phenotype is related to a defect within the MBP gene. Another dysmyelinating mutant allelic to *shi* (Bourre et al., 1980), called myelin deficient (*shi^mld*), has a slightly less severe phenotype, with reduced MBP in the CNS (Doolittle and Schweikart, 1972). Mice homozygous for the *shi^mld* allele have 5% of normal amounts of MBP at 30 days postnatal (Popko et al., 1987).

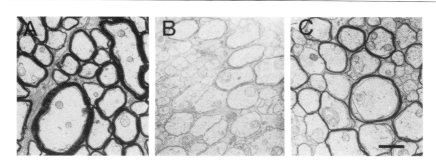

Figure 2. Electronmicrographs (modified from Readhead et al., 1987) of cross sections of optic nerve from a normal (A; +/+), a shiverer (B; *shi/shi*) and a transgenic shiverer mouse (C; *shi/shi;MBP^1/MBP^1*). Bar= 1μm.

The MBPs are a class of proteins that comprise 30% of the protein in CNS myelin (Lees and Brostoff, 1984) and may function to stabilize the close apposition of the cytoplasmic faces of compacted oligodendrocytic membrane (Martenson, 1981). Four major forms of MBP with molecular weights of 21.5, 18.5, 17.0, and 14.5 kilodaltons are present in mice (Barbarese et al., 1977). A single gene of about 32 kilobases in length and consisting of 7 exons codes for all four forms by differential splicing (Fig. 3; de Ferra et al., 1985). A recent report provides evidence for two additional exons that code for additional forms of MBP at much lower abundances (Newman et al., 1989). Mapping of the *shi* MBP gene revealed that the deletion spans a region from the second intron to several kilobases 3' to the last exon, and removes 5 of the 7 exons of the gene (Fig. 3; Roach et al., 1985; Molineaux et al., 1986). Without a full length gene it is impossible to code for normal MBP and this suggests that the MBP deficit is the primary cause for the severe hypomyelination observed in *shi* CNS.

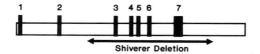

Figure 3. Diagram of MBP gene. The seven exons
encompasses about 32 kilobases of DNA. The *shi* deletion
encompasses a region from the second intron to several
kilobases 3' past the last exon.

The hypothesis that deficient MBP expression causes
dysmyelination in *shi* mice was proven when the phenotype was
partially reversed by introducing a cloned MBP gene into the
shi germline with transgenic techniques (Readhead et al.,
1987). A cosmid containing the full length mouse MBP gene
plus about 4 kilobases of 5' flanking DNA and 1 kilobase of
3' DNA was introduced into the germ line of a wild type
mouse and crossed onto the *shi* background. When *shi* mice
were bred with two copies of the transgene
(*shi/shi*;*MBP^1/MBP^1*) they did not shiverer or convulse and
lived normal life spans. However, unlike animals
heterozygous for the mutation (+/*shi*) that appear normal,
mice heterozygous for the transgene (*shi/shi*;*MBP^1/-*)
continued shivering and seizing throughout their lives.
Thus, the transgene had the capacity to contravene the
dysmyelinating phenotype, but was required in double dosage.
By contrast, a single copy of the wild type allele, as in
+/*shi* mice, suffices to allow expression of a normal
phenotype.

Tissue and developmental expression of the transgene
was similar to normal gene expression. Only RNA isolated
from brain contained MBP mRNA and expression peaked in
transgenic animals at postnatal day 18 (Readhead et al.,
1987) as in wild type animals (Carson et al., 1983). All
four forms of the protein were expressed in transgenic mice.
Hence, the 37 kilobase DNA fragment introduced into *shi* mice
contained sufficient code to direct appropriate temporal and
spacial expression of the gene besides coding for the
proteins. As implied by the lesser efficiency of the
transgene compared to the wild type gene, animals with two
copies of the transgene (*shi/shi*;*MBP^1/MBP^1*) expressed MBP
mRNA at approximately 25% of wild type levels and MBP at
relatively less amounts (Table 1). The reduced expression
of the *MBP^1* gene diminished, in turn, the oligodendrocytes'

ability to produce myelin in transgenic mice. The number of myelinated axons and the amount of myelin was much less than what was seen in the normal optic nerve (Fig. 2) and several axons were wrapped with loose layers of uncompacted membrane (Fig. 4).

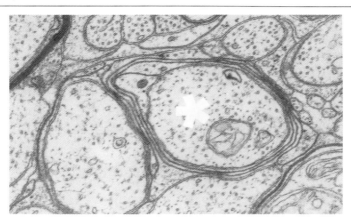

Figure 4. Electronmicrograph of axon (white star) with several wraps of oligodendrocyte membrane but no compacted myelin in an optic nerve of a mouse with an MBP gene dose of 12.5% of normal ($shi/shi;MBP^1/-$).

The ability to breed mice with genotypes that include normal, shi, shi^{mld} and MBP^1 genes provided a means to measure the influence of MBP expression on myelin formation. Possible gene combinations and the predicted gene doses based upon the measured mRNA and protein expression in the CNS of mice with genotypes given in Table 1 (Readhead et al., 1987) are listed in Table 2. Gene dose is defined as the percent of mRNA expressed relative to the normal value of 100%.

When values for MBP expression from the predicted gene doses listed in Table 2 are compared to the accumulation of MBP in the developing brain, most are equivalent to amounts expressed during early myelinogenesis (Fig. 1). If myelin formation is tightly coordinated with MBP expression, adult mice with genotypes coding for MBP levels similar to those of normally seen in early periods of myelinogenesis would be expected to produce myelin that is likewise equivalent in quantity and quality to that obtained in early periods of development. To test this hypothesis a detailed morphometric analysis was performed on electronmicrographs of CNS tissue. The aim was to measure the effect of reduced MBP expression on myelin parameters in mature mice with genotypes listed in Table 2.

TABLE 1. MBP mRNA and protein measured in normal, mutant, and transgenic mice. Values represent percent of normal.

Genotype	mRNA	Protein
shi/shi	0	<0.3
shi/shi;MBP[1]/-	12.5	8.5
shi/shi;MBP[1]/MBP[1]	25	20.6
+/+	100	100

TABLE 2. MBP gene doses for selected genotypes. Values are percent of normal and are predicted from values in Table 1.

Genotype	Gene Dose
shi/shi	0
shi[mld]/shi[mld]	5
shi/shi;MBP[1]/-	12.5
shi/shi[mld];MBP[1]/-	17.5
shi/shi;MBP[1]/MBP[1]	25
+/shi	50
+/shi;MBP[1]/-	62.5
+/+	100

METHODS

Optic nerves from mice with genotypes listed in Table 2 were prepared for electron microscopy at 60 days after birth (except for *shi[mld]/shi[mld]* which were prepared at 30 days postnatal) by double aldehyde perfusion, OsO_4 postfixation and Epon embedding. Data were collected from electronmicrographic prints at 30,000x magnification of thin

cross sections of the optic nerves of each mouse with a
morphometric analysis system consisting of a Jandel
Scientific (Corte Madera, CA) digitizing tablet and a Dell
(Austin, TX) 310 microcomputer running Jandel Sigma Scan
software. Axon circumference and area were measured, and
the numbers of myelinated, unmyelinated, and wrapped axons
were counted. On average, 800 axons were measured for each
sample. Percent drift frequency analysis (Bronson et al.,
1978) verified that the samples were sufficient to represent
the total population of axons in each optic nerve.

RESULTS

Percentage of Myelinated Axons is Linked to MBP Expression.

As predicted from the developmental data in Figure 1
the greater the degree of MBP expression the greater the
percentage of myelinated axons in the optic nerve (Fig. 5).
The largest increments in the percentages of unmyelinated
and myelinated axons were apparent in the gene dose range
between 0% and 50% corresponding in the normal case to the
early period of myelinogenesis, when oligodendrocytes are
rapidly increasing their MBP expression and myelin membrane
formation.

The percentage of axons that had several wraps of
oligodendrocytic membrane but no compacted myelin (Fig. 4)
peaked at 17.5% gene dose. This peak matched a shoulder on
the unmyelinated curve. A presence of wrapped axons in mice
with low gene doses (5% to 25%) may represent a condition in
which MBP expression is sufficient to elicit a deposition of
myelin membrane by oligodendrocytes but not adequate for
formation of compacted myelin.

Myelin Thickness is Linked to MBP Expression.

As the *shi* mouse genome acquired more MBP gene activity
the average thickness of myelin increased. Figure 6 shows
the distribution of myelin thickness of myelinated axons
averaged for animals with low gene doses (12.5%, 17.5%, 25%)
that correspond to the steep rise in MBP expression and
myelin formation during early development, and for animals
with high doses (50%, 62.5%, 100%) corresponding to the

situation in adult CNS. The average myelin thickness in low
dose mice was significantly less than average myelin

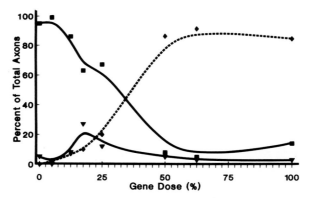

Figure 5. Percent of myelinated (◆), unmyelinated (■),
and "wrapped" (▲) axons counted in the optic nerves of mice
with various genotypes that give MBP gene doses ranging from
0% to 100%. Computer generated best fit curves are
superimposed upon the data points.

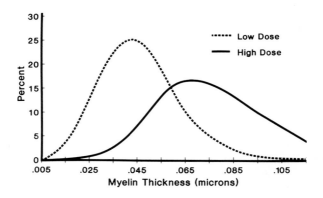

Figure 6. Distribution of myelin thickness in optic nerves
of mice with low doses of MBP gene (pooled 12.5%, 17.5%,
25%) and high doses (pooled 50%, 62.5%, 100%).

thickness in high dose mice. These data suggest that as the expression of MBP is increased, oligodendrocytes lay down more lamellae around axons as well as increase the number of axons that they myelinate.

Selection of Axons to Myelinate is Linked to MBP Expression.

A comparison of axon circumference with gene dose revealed that the mean myelinated axon caliber in animals with low MBP gene doses was larger than in mice with higher doses (Table 3). This negative correlation suggests that with limited MBP resources, oligodendrocytes preferentially choose to myelinate axons with larger axon circumferences. As the amount of MBP available to oligodendrocytes increases they interact with axons of progressively smaller caliber.

TABLE 3. Circumference of myelinated axons versus MBP gene dose. Values of gene dose are percent of normal. Values for axon circumference are μm ± standard error.

Genotype	Gene Dose	Axon Circum.
$shi/shi;MBP^1/-$	12.5	3.38 ±0.13
$shi/shi^{mld};MBP^1/-$	17.5	3.17 ±0.21
$shi/shi;MBP^1/MBP^1$	25	3.13 ±0.08
$+/shi$	50	2.86 ±0.04
$+/shi;MBP^1/-$	62.5	2.94 ±0.05
$+/+$	100	2.55 ±0.04

CONCLUSION

In summary, oligodendrocytes in mice with partially reconstituted *shi* genomes mimicked their counterparts' behavior in the normally developing nervous system. As the oligodendrocytes acquired, by one means or another, the capacity to express greater amounts of MBP more axons were myelinated, thicker myelin was formed and smaller axons were included in the myelinated axon pool. We have shown this quantitatively in adult mice with various MBP genotypes, and similar data are available for the normal developing optic nerve (Tennekoon et al., 1977). During the first few postnatal days an increase the expression of MBP by oligodendrocytes is mirrored by an increase in the rate of myelin formation. More axons join the myelinated axon pool and more wrappings of membrane are added to the thickness of the myelin sheath.

The Myelin Basic Proteins are conventionally viewed as structural components of the myelin membrane. Our data, indicating that oligodendroglia membrane-forming activity varies in proportion to the extent of MBP synthesis, suggest a far more dynamic role for these proteins in modulating the developmental behavior of the oligodendroglia cell. It remains to be explored whether certain of the MBPs, which are synthesized at different rates during development (Barbarese et al., 1978), might be more important than other ones in this dynamic interplay.

It appears that reconstituting the *shi* genome with genes expressing MBP at less than normal levels is reflected in adult oligodendrocytes that function as if they were immature cells. It could be said that in terms of oligodendrocytic function these mice have the CNS of a neonatal animal carried in the body of an adult.

ACKNOWLEDGEMENTS

We would like to thank Patrick Enos, Elaine Gwosdz and Marcia Lind for their excellent technical assistance. This work was supported by NIH grants HD18655, NS20820, and AG07687 and funds from the Retina Research Foundation. A portion of this work was performed in the Alice R. McPherson Laboratory of Retinal Research.

REFERENCES

Barbarese E, Braun PE, Carson JH (1977). Identification of prelarge and presmall basic proteins in mouse myelin and their structural relationship to large and small basic protein. Proc Natl Acad Sci USA 74:3360-3364.
Barbarese E, Carson JH, Braun PE (1978). Accumulation of the four myelin basic proteins in mouse brain during development. J Neurochem 31:779-782.

Barnett F, Davisson M, Villa-Komaroff L, Sidman RL, Shine HD (1985). Localization of mouse MBP gene to chromosome 18 by *in situ* hybridization. Trans Am Soc Neurochem 16:196.

Biddle F, March E, Miller JR (1973). Research news. Mouse News Lett 48:24.

Bronson RT, Bishop Y, Hedley-White ET (1978). A contribution to the electron microscopic morphometric analysis of peripheral nerve. J Comp Neurol 178:177-186.

Carson JH, Nielson ML, Barbarese E (1983). Developmental regulation of myelin basic protein expression in mouse brain. Dev Biol 96:485-492.

de Ferra F, Engh H, Hudson L, Kamholz J, Puckett C, Molineaux S, Lazzarini RA (1985) Alternative splicing accounts for the four forms of myelin basic protein. Cell 43:721-727.

Doolittle DP, Schweikart KM (1977). Myelin deficient, a new neurological mutant in the mouse. J Hered 68:331-332.

Dupouey P, Jacque C, Bourre JM, Cesselin F, Privat A, Baumann N (1979). Immunochemical studies of myelin basic protein in shiverer mouse devoid of major dense line of myelin. Neurosci Lett 12:113-118.

Kirschner DA, Ganser AL (1980). Compact myelin exists in the absence of basic protein in the shiverer mutant mouse. Nature 283:207-210.

Lees MB, Brostoff SW (1984). Proteins of myelin. In Morell P (ed): "Myelin," New York: Plenum Press, pp 197-224.

Martenson RE (1981) Prediction of the secondary structure of myelin basic protein. J Neurochem 36:1543-1560.

Molineaux SM, Engh H, de Ferra F, Hudson L, Lazzarini RA (1986). Recombination within the myelin basic protein gene created the dysmyelinating shiverer mouse mutation. Proc Natl Acad Sci USA 83:7542-7546.

Newman S, Kiamura K, Campagnoni C, Campagnoni AT (1989). Expression of two novel exons of the mouse MBP gene. Trans Am Soc Neurochem 20:144.

Norton WT, Poduslo SE (1973). Myelination in rat brain: changes in myelin composition during brain maturation. J Neuochem 21:759-773.

Popko B, Puckett C, Lai E, Shine HD, Readhead C, Takahashi N, Hunt SW, Sidman RL, Hood L (1987). Myelin deficient mice: expression of myelin basic protein and generation of mice with varying levels of myelin. Cell 48:713-721.

Readhead C, Popko B, Takahashi N, Shine HD, Saavedra RA, Sidman RL, Hood L (1987). Expression of a myelin basic protein gene in transgenic shiverer mice: correction of the dysmyelinating phenotype. Cell 48:703-712.

Roach A, Takahashi N, Pravtcheva D, Ruddle F, Hood L (1985) Chromosomal mapping of mouse myelin basic protein gene and structure and transcription of the partially deleted gene in shiverer mutant mice. Cell 42:149-155.

Rosenbluth J (1980). Peripheral myelin in the mouse mutant shiverer. J Comp Neurol 193:729-739.

Sidman RL, Conover CS, Carson JH (1985). Shiverer gene maps near the distal end of chromosome 18 in the house mouse. Cytogenet Cell Genet 39:241-245.

Tennekoon GI, Cohen SR, Price DL, McKhann GM (1977). Myelinogenesis in optic nerve. J Cell Biol 72:604-616.

Dynamic Interactions of Myelin Proteins, pages 93–108

MYELIN BASIC PROTEIN, MHC RESTRICTION MOLECULES AND T CELL REPERTOIRE

Arthur A. Vandenbark, George Hashim and Halina Offner
Departments of Neurology (A.A.V. and H.O.) and Immunology and Microbiology (A.A.V.), Oregon Health Sciences University, Portland, Oregon 97201, and St. Luke's/Roosevelt Hospital and Columbia University (G.H.), New York, NY

INTRODUCTION

T cell recognition of antigen involves interaction of the T cell receptor complex with immunogenic peptides which are cleaved from the antigen during processing and expressed in association with Class I or Class II major histocompatibility molecules (MHC) (Unanue and Allen, 1987; Watts and McConnell, 1987). It is now widely held that the extracellular domains of each MHC allele form a single peptide binding site which associates preferentially with amino acid sequences sharing a common motif which may mimic and displace an internal ligand within the MHC molecule (Buus et al., 1987; Guillet et al., 1987). Regions of the peptide that are not involved in MHC binding are available for interaction with the T cell receptor complex (Margalit et al., 1987; Rothbard and Taylor, 1988). Peptides which bind strongly to the MHC molecule are likely to be immunogenic, whereas those which bind poorly are not (Buus et al., 1987; Guillet et al., 1987; Margalit et al., 1987; Rothbard and Taylor, 1988; Babbitt et al., 1985). Thus T cell responses to a given molecule are limited to epitopes which associate preferentially with the available MHC molecules.

It is probable that these principles govern T helper cell recognition of the autoantigen myelin basic protein (MBP). Under normal conditions, this central nervous system protein is found in association with the internal myelin membrane, where it is thought to function as a self-adhesive molecule which keeps the myelin membrane tightly wrapped against itself around the axon (Brady et al., 1981;

Moscarello et al., 1986). Through natural catabolism, low
levels of MBP are present in cerebrospinal fluid (CSF),
usually without immunological consequences. Increased
concentrations of BP and BP-like fragments in CSF or urine
are indicative of periods of active demyelination (Whitaker
and Snyder, 1982). In the context of an inflammatory
response, however, MBP is highly immunogenic and widely
encephalitogenic.

Immunization of animals with MBP results in the
development of EAE (Alvord, 1984), a paralytic and often
demyelinating disease mediated by T helper lymphocytes which
express receptors for one or more immunodominant epitopes on
the MBP molecule (Vandenbark et al., 1985a; Bourdette et
al., 1988; Sakai et al., 1988). Encephalitogenic epitopes
are different for each animal strain, and are influenced by
the available Class II MHC molecules, predominantly I-A,
expressed by antigen presenting cells (APC) (Bourdette et
al., 1988; Sakai et al., 1988; Beraud et al., 1986; Zamvil
et al., 1985; Offner et al., 1986). Studies in F1 animals
have shown that in the presence of both parental MHC types,
only one epitope/MHC combination predominates, suggesting a
hierarchy of immunodominance (Beraud et al., 1986; Zamvil et
al., 1985).

MBP-specific T helper lymphocyte lines selected with
whole GP-BP could induce EAE in Lewis rats (Vandenbark et
al., 1985b; Ben-Nun and Cohen, 1982). These lines recognized only the Lewis rat encephalitogenic determinant contained in residues 69-89 of guinea pig MBP (Vandenbark et
al., 1985; Offner et al., 1987), and all other T cell specificities present in the immunized lymph node population
were lost during the in vitro selection procedure. The
focused recognition of the 69-89 determinant by the T cell
line raised the possibility that there was limited heterogeneity among T cell clones within the line. In this chapter, we describe the fine specificity, MHC restriction, T
cell receptor V gene use, encephalitogenicity, and regulation of T cells responsive to the 69-89 determinant of BP.

DEFINITION OF ENCEPHALITOGENIC T CELL EPITOPES

The encephalitogenic T cell epitope for Lewis rats was
defined in detail using synthetic peptides that corresponded
to overlapping sequences within the 69-89 region of guinea

pig (GP-) (GSLPQKSQRSQDENPVVHF) and rat (Rt-)
(GSLPQKSQRTQDENPVVHF) BP. T cell lines were selected to GP-
BP as we described previously (Vandenbark et al., 1985b). T
cell clones responsive to GP-BP were obtained from partially
selected lines using the soft agar technique (Chou et al.,
1988), and were evaluated for proliferation responses to
synthetic peptides. The peptide specificity for several
representative clones is presented in Table I. All of the
clones responded best to the S72-89 sequence of GP-BP, and
all were encephalitogenic. Other sequences, including the
S72-84 and S75-89 peptides were less stimulatory, and the
S69-81 and S75-84 sequences were unable to induce proliferation (Table 1). These results indicated that the 75-84
sequence contained the essential amino acids for T cell
recognition, but could not stimulate encephalitogenic T
cells without the addition of residues 72-74 or 85-89.

Table 1.   Response of GP-BP Specific T Cell Clones

CPM/1000

Clone	S69-81	S72-89	S72-84	S75-89	EAE
C11	0	14	7	3	+
C12	0	55	31	3	+
C13	0	26	12	3	+
C14	0	91	47	17	+
C15	0	75	36	7	+
C16	0	46	21	3	+
C17	0	36	24	4	+

Immunization of Lewis rats with the Rt 72-84 sequence
(Rt-S55S) produced a T cell line that responded initially to
the S72-84 and S72-89 peptides, but were nearly unresponsive
to Rt- or GP-BP (Offner et al., 1988). T cell clones selected from the Rt-S55S line at hat point had two distinct
patterns of response: Clones that recognized the BP and the
S55S peptide adoptively transferred delayed type hypersensitivity (not shown) and EAE (Table 2). The clones also

recognized residues 69-81, but not peptide 75-89. In contrast, T cell clones that responded only to synthetic peptide Rt-S55S but not to the parent BP adoptively transferred DTH (not shown) but not EAE (Table 2). The same clones failed to respond to either the S69-81 or S75-89 peptides (Table 2). These results indicated that the encephalitogenic Rt-S55S sequence housed a minimum of two T cell epitopes with differing specificities and functions. One epitope was immunodominant and resembled the encephalitogenic region of the intact BP molecule. The second non-encephalitogenic epitope was restricted to the S55S sequence and was not shared by the parent BP, the S69-81 or the S75-89 sequences. Both types of Rt-S55S-specific clones differed in fine specificity from encephalitogenic clones selected from GP-BP immunized rats, indicating that uniformity of T cell recognition of the encephalitogenic epitope is not an absolute condition for T cells to be encephalitogenic. Of general importance, these data showed that more than one T cell specificity could be encephalitogenic in Lewis rats.

Table 2.   Response of Rt-S72-84 Specific T Cell Clones

	CPM/1000				
Clone	S69-81	S72-89	Rt-S72-84	S75-89	EAE
D	34	25	52	0	+
G	13	37	56	0	+
E	0	0	37	0	-
H	0	0	28	0	-
I	0	0	49	0	-
J	0	0	40	0	-

ANALYSIS OF T CELL RECEPTOR GENES

Prospects for specific immune intervention in T-cell mediated autoimmune disease by anti-idiotype regulation depend on the degree of diversity of the responder cell

antigen-receptor repertoire. We were struck by the similarity in fine specificity and encephalitogenic activity of
Lewis rat T cell clones responsive to the 72-89 sequence of
GP-BP, and upon further analysis, we found that these T
cells used a limited set of T-cell receptor V genes (Happ et
al., 1988; Burns et al., 1989). Furthermore, using cloned T
cell receptor α and β chain cDNAs from a hybrid specific for
the 72-89 sequence of Rt-BP, we found that the encephalitogenic T cell clones all used the same Vβ chain (with sequence homology to the mouse Vβ8.2 family) and 70% the same
Vα chain (with sequence homology to the mouse Vα2 family) in
their T cell receptor (summarized in Table III). In contrast, encephalitogenic T cells responding to the Rt-S55S
determinant on Rt-BP (72-84 sequence) did not utilize the
same Vα or Vβ genes in their T cell receptor (Table 3).
These results demonstrate that restricted V gene usage
involving the Vβ8.2 and Vα2 families occurs in response to
the primary immunodominant epitope of GP-BP. However, these
V genes are not the only combination that can be utilized to
produce an encephalitogenic T cell response the Lewis rat.

Table 3.   T Cell Receptor V Gene Use

T Cell Specificity	Restriction	Encephalitogenic	Vα 2	Vβ 8.2
72-89 (GP)	I-A	+	+	+
72-89 (Rt)	I-A	+	+	+
72-84 (Rt)	I-A	+ or -	-	-

LYMPHOCYTE VACCINATION

    Restricted V gene usage provides a basis for observed
idiotypic regulation of autoreactive T-cells, and possible
therapy for autoimmune disease. One approach for inducing
immunologic recognition and possible regulation of encephalitogenic T cells is to vaccinate naive animals with T
cells which have been attenuated by hydrostatic pressure
treatment or crosslinking of cell surface molecules. We
evaluated several vaccination protocols for their ability to
induce resistance to EAE in the Lewis rat (Vandenbark et
al., 1987; Vandenbark et al., 1987). Both clinical and

histologic signs of active EAE could be prevented by vac-
cinating three times with attenuated BP specific T cell
lines or a BP specific T cell clone, but not with a PPD
specific T cell line (Fig. 1). In contrast, protection
against passive EAE appeared to be clonotypic, since vaccination with the clone but not BP line cells induced complete resistance to clone but not BP line-mediated EAE (Fig.
1). Vaccination induced delayed type hypersensitivity (DTH)
reactions against autologous T cells, mostly to shared antigens. These results confirmed the validity of using lymphocyte vaccination to regulate pernicious T cells and delinea-
ted conditions and restrictions involved in the vaccination
protocols. Although the target autoantigen on the T cell
surface has not been identified, we suspect it to be the T
cell receptor itself, since this would account for clonotypic regulation.

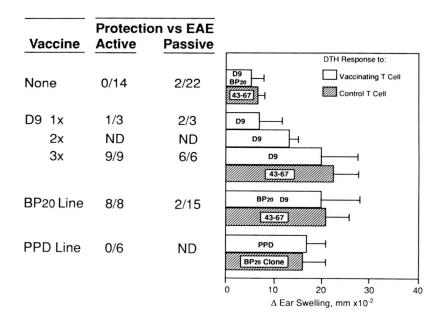

Vaccine	Protection vs EAE	
	Active	Passive
None	0/14	2/22
D9 1x	1/3	2/3
2x	ND	ND
3x	9/9	6/6
BP20 Line	8/8	2/15
PPD Line	0/6	ND

Figure 1. Lymphocyte vaccination induces protection against
EAE and DTH reactions against attenuated T lymphocytes.
Rats were vaccinated with antigen activated, hydrostatic
pressure-treated (1,300 ATM) and irradiated (2,500 R) T
cells. One week later, the rats were ear tested with

HUMAN T CELL RESPONSES TO MYELIN BASIC PROTEIN

The regulation of BP epitope-specific T cells by
vaccination has potential application to human autoimmune
diseases that involve restricted T cell repertoires.
Multiple sclerosis (MS) is characterized by inflammatory
lesions and demyelination of the central nervous system, and
motor dysfunction, and has some similarity to EAE. Addi-
tionally, MS has both a genetic predisposition (increased
occurrence of HLA-DR2 relative to the neurologically un-
affected population) and immunologic abnormalities (Waksman
and Reynolds, 1984). Responses to BP in MS patients have
been difficult to observe, but if an encephalitogenic process is involved in the pathogenesis of MS, BP should be
considered as one of the possible target antigens. In the
event that human BP responses involve a restricted T cell
repertoire, it would be feasible to test the hypothesis that
BP is involved in the pathogenesis of disease by eliminating
BP-specific T cells (i.e., by vaccination).

We have analyzed the response of human T cells
(Vandenbark et al., in press; Chou et al., in press) to MBP.
Using several different MBP preparations to enhance the
probability of detecting significant proliferation responses
of blood lymphocytes, we screened 26 normal donors, 27
patients with MS, and 20 patients with other neurological
diseases (OND). Although the level of proliferation was
rather modest, we found that blood cells from MS patients
responded significantly to human BP, compared with neurologically normal donors (Fig. 2). The rate of positive
responses in the MS patient group was also significantly
greater (78%) than normal donors (31%), with an intermediate
rate of response (45%) in patients with other neurological
diseases (OND) (Table 4). These results indicate that the
immunological recognition of BP is more prevalent in humans,

300,000 activated and irradiated T cells of the same or
different specificities, as indicated within the bars of the
graph. Delayed type hypersensitivity was measured as the
maximum increase in ear swelling after 24-48 hours. Error
bars indicate the S.D. Active or passive EAE was induced
one week after the DTH reaction was administered. Numbers
indicate animals protected versus animals challenged with
EAE.

especially in MS patients, than was previously suspected.
The increased T cell responses observed suggest the
increased probability of encephalitogenic T cell
specificities.

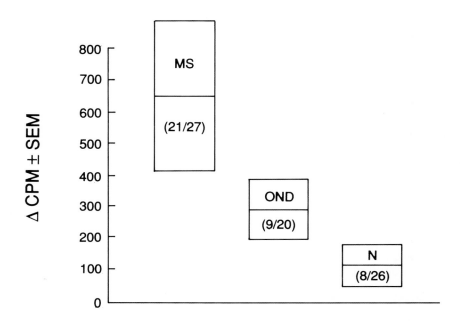

Figure 2.   Lymphocyte proliferation responses of blood mono-
nuclear cells to human BP.   Each bar represents the mean ±
S.E.M. of the net proliferation response (CPM in the presence of BP minus CPM in the presence of medium alone).
Numbers in parentheses indicate the number of patients with
significant counts over background versus the total number
tested.   The magnitude of response of MS patients as a group
was significantly greater than that of normal donors (p <
0.01).   The background CPM response for each group was:
900 ± 109 (n = 26) for normal subjects; 929 ± 141 (n = 27)
for MS patients; 846 ± 106 (n = 20) for OND patients.

Table 4.　　　　　　　Human BP Responses

N	MS	OND
8/26	21/27	9/20
(31%)	(78%)	(45%)

The identification of predominant epitopes of human BP and a better knowledge of how the MHC molecules influence the pattern of T cell responsiveness may provide insights into differences in BP responses among patients and normal donors. We found that the modest response of blood cells to BP was essential for the selection of human BP-specific T cell lines (Vandenbark et al., in press and Table 5). From positive donors, we selected 14 human MBP-specific T cell lines (using techniques similar to those for rat T cell lines), and characterized both the immunodominant T cell epitopes and associated MHC restriction molecules (Chou et al., in press). Responses to MBP fragments 1-38 and 44-89 were of higher magnitude and frequency in MS patients than in normals, although response to P4 was not different (Fig. 3). HLA-DR was used predominantly to restrict the T cell responses (Table 6). HLA-DQ was used much less frequently, but only in patients with MS or OND.

Table 5.　　　　　　　T Cell Line Selection

Stim #	C	HBP	1-38	44-89	%-170	HSV
1 PBL	1 ± 0	3 ± 0	---	---	---	9 ± 1
2 APC	1 ± 0	15 ± 2	6 ± 2	2 ± 0	11 ± 3	1 ± 1
3 APC	0 ± 0	14 ± 1	7 ± 1	2 ± 0	14 ± 1	0 ± 1

underline = significantly greater than control.

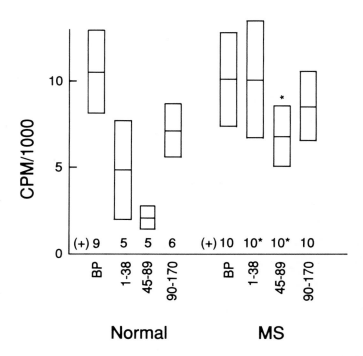

Figure 3. BP-specific T cell line proliferation to fragments of BP. Each bar represents the mean CPM ± S.E.M. of
the net proliferation response (CPM/1000 ^{3}H-thymidine uptake) of 20,000 T cells stimulated with 10-50 µg of each of
human BP or BP fragments presented by autologous monocytes.
Asterisks indicate significant differences in CPM (for
fragment containing residues 45-89) between MS patients and
normal donors, and significant differences in the frequency
of responses between the groups to the 1-38 and 45-89
fragments. No differences in response to whole human BP or
to fragment 90-170 were observed.

Table 6.   Number of Patients Using Each Locus for Response
(# of responses)

	MS	N	OND	TOTAL
DR	7/7 (19)	3/4 (3)	1/1 (4)	11/12 (26)
DQ	4/7 (5)	0/4 (0)	1/1 (1)	5/12 (6)
DP	0/7 (0)	1/4 (1)	0/1 (0)	1/12 (1)

The four normal T cell lines recognized predominantly single separate epitopes restricted by HLA-DR or -DP molecules, whereas the MS and OND lines recognized multiple epitopes restricted by HLA-DR or -DQ molecules (Table 7).   In total, at least eight different T cell epitopes were identified on human MBP (Table 7).   HLA-DR2, which is in linkage disequilibrium in MS patients, was unusual in that it could restrict multiple epitopes, suggesting that its association with various MBP peptides is not stringent.   These data raise the possibility that HLA-DR2 may be involved in presenting a wide variety of MBP epitopes, thus increasing the chances of inducing an encephalitogenic T cell response. The complex pattern of response to MBP in patients suggests greater sensitization to this widely encephalitogenic molecule, and perhaps is related to the disease process itself. These data (summarized in Fig. 4) provide the first evidence of genetically restricted human T cell recognition of MBP, and constitute a new approach to illuminate the genetic basis of autoimmunity against CNS tissue.

Table 7.   <u>MHC Restriction of Epitopes Recognized by T Cells</u>

Class II Locus/Allele	N	MS	OND
DR2	96-117 (2)	45-59 (59-74)(3) (75-89) (87-99) (118-157)(2)	1-38 28-42 87-99 96-117
DR3	87-99	- - -	- - -
DR4	- - -	1-38(2) 87-99 118-157	- - -
DR5	- - -	1-38(2) 87-99(2)	- - -
DQw1	- - -	1-28 (59-74) 96-117(2)	96-117
DQw3	- - -	118-157	- - -
DP	1-38	- - -	- - -

Figure 4.   <u>Summary</u>

MS patients had increased frequency of BP responses.

BP specific T cell lines only from responders:

 * Increased MS response to P1 and P2.

 * Restricted predominantly by HLA-DR.

 * HLA-DQ restriction only in patients.

 * Multiple BP-peptide associations with HLA-DR2.

SUMMARY AND CONCLUSIONS

Our laboratory has developed a broad base of information in rats and mice describing the properties of encephalitogenic T cells. Using the T cell line selection technique to identify dominant T cell specificities, we were the first to identify new encephalitogenic epitopes and MHC restriction molecules in the Lewis rat and the SJL mouse. Furthermore, using the soft agar technique, we have isolated encephalitogenic Lewis rat T cell clones specific for defined synthetic epitopes of BP. With our colleagues, we have identified and sequenced the V region genes, and deduced the amino acid sequence of proteins which these clones use preferentially in their T cell receptor. Furthermore, we have successfully induced protection against EAE by the lymphocyte vaccination approach, using attenuated encephalitogenic T cells as the vaccine.

Using this information, we have made significant progress in characterizing and understanding human T lymphocyte responses to BP. Recent results indicate that MBP reactivity is more frequent in MS patients than in controls, suggesting a greater degree of sensitization, and a potential involvement of BP as a target antigen. Since human BP responses also appear to be directed at immunodominant epitopes (as we have observed in rodents), it is probable that human T cells will also use preferential combinations of T cell receptor V genes. The ability to induce specific regulation or removal of autoreactive T cells will allow for the first time an assessment of cause and effect in human diseases. Immunoregulation directed at the TCR polypeptides may allow selective suppression of encephalitogenic clones, and may have direct application in human diseases such as MS, or in other autoimmune situations where preferential TCR V gene usage can be identified.

Future Prospects

* Disease-related BP epitopes?

* Testing of encephalitogenicity in SCID-Hu mice

* TCR V gene usage in P1 and P2 specific clones

* Selective regulation of T cell clones using common TCR V genes

ACKNOWLEDGEMENTS

The authors wish to thank Drs. Yuan Chou, Margarita Vainiene, Ruth Whitham, Dennis Bourdette, Richard Jones, Bozena Celnik, John Chilgren, Ellen Heber-Katz, Selene Chou and Greg Konat for their contributions to the work described above. This work was supported by the Veterans Administration, and by NIH grants NS23221, NS23444, and NS21466.

REFERENCES

Alvord EC Jr (1984). In Alvord EC Jr, Kies M, Suckling A (eds): Experimental Allergic Encephalomyelitis: A useful model for Multiple Sclerosis. New York: Alan R. Liss, Inc., pp 523.

Babbitt BP, Allen PM, Matsueda G, Haber E, Unanue ER (1985). Binding of immunogenic peptides to Ia histocompatibility molecules. Nature (London) 317:359-361.

Ben-Nun A, Cohen IR (1982). Experimental autoimmune encephalomyelitis (EAE) mediated by cell lines: Process of selection of lines and characterization of the cells. J Immunol 129:303.

Beraud E, Reshef T, Vandenbark AA, Offner H, Fritz R, Chou C-HJ, Bernard D, Cohen IR (1986). Experimental autoimmune encephalomyelitis mediated by T lymphocyte lines: Genotype of antigen presenting cells influences immunodominant epitope of basic protein. J Immunol 136:511-515.

Bourdette DN, Vandenbark AA, Meshul C, Whitham R, Offner H (1988). Basic protein specific T cell lines that induce experimental autoimmune encephalomyelitis in SJL/J mice: Comparison with Lewis rat lines. Cell Immunol 112:351-363.

Brady GW, Fein DB, Wood DD, Moscarello MA (1981). The interaction of basic proteins from normal and multiple sclerosis myelin with phosphatidylglycerol vesicles. FEBS Letters 125:159-160.

Burns FR, Li X, Shen N, Offner H, Chou Y, Vandenbark AA, Heber-Katz E (1989). Both rat and mouse T cell receptors specific for the encephalitogenic determinant of myelin basic protein use similar $V\alpha$ and $V\beta$ chain genes even though the major histocompatibility complex and encephalitogenic determinants being recognized are different. J Exp Med 169:27-39.

Buus S, Sette A, Colon SM, Miles C, Grey HM (1987). The relation between major histocompatibility complex (MHC) restriction and the capacity of Ia to bind immunogenic peptides. Science 235:1353-1358.

Chou YK, Vandenbark AA, Jones RE, Hashim G, Offner H (1988, in press). Selection of encephalitogenic rat T lymphocyte clones recognizing an immunodominant epitope on myelin basic protein. J Neurosci Res.

Chou YK, Vainiene M, Whitham R, Bourdette D, Chou CH-J, Hashim GA, Offner H, Vandenbark AA (in press). Response of human T lymphocytes to myelin basic protein: Association of dominant epitopes with HLA Class II restriction molecules. J Neurosci Res.

Guillet J-G, Lai M-Z, Briner TJ, Buus S, Sette A, Grey HM, Smith JA, Gefter ML (1987). Immunological Self, nonself discrimination. Science 235:865-870.

Happ MP, Kiraly AS, Offner H, Vandenbark AA, Heber-Katz E (1988). The autoreactive T cell population in experimental allergic encephalomyelitis: T cell receptor β chain rearrangements. J Neuroimmunol 19:191-204.

Margalit H, Spouge JL, Cornette JL, Ease KB, DeLisi C, Bersofsky JA (1987). Prediction of immunodominant helper T cell antigenic sites from the primary sequence. J Immunol 138(7):2213.

Moscarello MA, Brady GW, Fein DB, Wood DD, Cruz TF (1986). The role of charge microheterogeneity of basic protein in the formation and maintenance of the multilayered structure of myelin: a possible role in multiple sclerosis. J Neurosci Res 15:87-99.

Offner H, Brostoff SW, Vandenbark AA (1986). Antibodies against I-A and I-E determinants inhibit the in vitro activation of an encephalitogenic T lymphocyte line. Cell Immunol 100:364-373.

Offner H, Hashim GA, Vandenbark AA (1987). Response of rat encephalitogenic T lymphocyte lines to synthetic peptides of myelin basic protein. J Neurosci Res 17:344-348.

Offner H, Hashim GA, Chou YK, Celnik B, Jones R, Vandenbark AA (1988). Encephalitogenic T cell clones with variant receptor specificity. J Immunol 141:3828-3832.

Offner H, Jones R, Celnik B, Vandenbark AA (1989). Lymphocyte vaccination against experimental autoimmune encephalomyelitis: Evaluation of vaccination protocols. J Neuroimmunol 21:13-22.

Rothbard JB, Taylor WR (1988). A sequence pattern common to T cell epitopes. The EMBO Journal 7:93-100.

Sakai K, Sinha AA, Mitchell DJ, Zamvil SS, Rothbard JB, McDevitt HO, Steinman L (1988). Involvement of distinct murine T-cell receptors in the autoimmune encephalitogenic response to nested epitopes of myelin basic protein. Proc Natl Acad Sci USA 85:8608-8612.

Unanue ER, Allen PM (1987). The basis for the immunoregulatory role of macrophages and other accessory cells. Science 136:551.

Vandenbark AA, Offner H, Reshef T, Fritz R, Chou C, Cohen IR (1985a). Specificity of T lymphocyte lines specific for peptides of myelin basic protein. J Immunol 135(1):229.

Vandenbark AA, Gill T, Offner H (1985b). A myelin basic protein specific T lymphocyte line which mediates experimental autoimmune encephalomyelitis. J Immunol 135:223-228.

Vandenbark AA, Bourdette D, Whitham R, Offner H (1987). Regulation of epitope specific encephalitogenic T lymphocytes: Rationale for vaccination of multiple sclerosis patients. In Rose CF (ed): Proceedings of International Symposium on Multiple Sclerosis. London: John Libbey and Company Ltd., pp 27-33.

Vandenbark AA, Chou YK, Vainiene M, Chilgren J, Bourdette D, Whitham R, Chou CH-J, Konat G (in press). Human T lymphocyte response to myelin basic protein (MBP): Selection of T lymphocyte lines from MBP responsive donors. J Neurosci Res.

Waksman BH, Reynolds WE (1984). Multiple sclerosis as a disease of immune regulation. Proc Soc Exp Biol Med 175:282-294.

Watts TH, McConnell HM (1987). Biophysical aspects of antigen recognition by T cells. Ann Rev Immunol 5:461.

Whitaker JN, Snyder DS (1982). Myelin components in the cerebrospinal fluid in diseases affecting central nervous system myelin. Clin Allergy Immunol 2:469-482.

Zamvil SS, Nelson PA, Mitchell DJ, Knobler RL, Fritz RB, Steinman L (1985). Encephalitogenic T cell clones specific for myelin basic protein: An unusual bias in antigen recognition. J Exp Med 162:2107.

Dynamic Interactions of Myelin Proteins, pages 109–192
© 1990 Alan R. Liss, Inc.

ANTIBODIES TO THE MYELIN MEMBRANE

Eugene D. Day, Ph.D.

Professor Emeritus of Immunology
Duke University Medical Center
Durham, North Carolina

ANTIBODIES TO MYELIN BASIC PROTEIN (MBP) AND MBP PEPTIDES

(a) Introduction

Even though MBP is not one of the more immunogenic
myelin components, giving rise only to an antigen binding
capacity (ABC) of 5 μM under the best of circumstances in
hyperimmunized rabbits (where hyperimmunity ordinarily
would be expected to be 50 μM) and more usually to ABCs of
less than 750 nM in guinea pigs, rats and mice (as measured at 10 nM total MBP concentration), it has received
the greatest amount of immunological attention among myelin components because of its role in encephalitogenic
events. Anti-MBP antibodies, themselves, have not been
completely dissociated from the main immunological pathway
leading to EAE (1-3), interest in them remains high because of the multiple uses to which they have and will
continue to be put:

(i) mono- and polyclonal probes to help determine
primary, secondary, tertiary and even quaternary structures;

(ii) mono- and polyclonal probes to help establish
exposed structures and/or determinants;

(iii) regulatory molecules of immunological pathways
that may inhibit or aid demyelinating effector T cells;

(iv) reagents to help disclose shared determinants
between MBP and other tissue and viral components and
secretions through the avenue of cross-reaction studies;

(v)   reagents to measure metabolic fragments in body fluids associated with demyelinating disease processes;

(vi)   immunohistochemical (fluorescent, radioactive, enzyme-active) stains of myelin processes in developmental studies of brain, of oligodendroglial cells in cultures, and of pathological brain specimens;

(vii)   electron-dense labeled probes in electron microscopic investigations;

(viii)   affinity column chromatography;

(ix)   indicators of the genetics of the autoimmune response to MBP;

(x)   probes to study the roles of idiotypy and immune complexes in MBP-associated diseases.

(b)   Methods for the Measurement of Anti-MBP Antibodies

(i)   Classical methods for the detection and measurement of anti-MBP antibodies have not been too fruitful because of the weakness of most antisera; moreover, reactions that have been recorded have largely been confined to rabbit antisera. A quantitative precipitin reaction between bovine MBP and a rabbit antiserum has been demonstrated;[4] immunodiffusion reactions between a number of MBPs and rabbit anti-chicken MBP have been photographed;[5,6] immunoelectrophoretic patterns have been developed for rabbit anti-rabbit MBP antisera[5] as well as rabbit antisera against canine and porcine MBPs;[7] and a quantitative microcomplement fixation analysis of rabbit anti-human MBP with human, monkey, and guinea pig MBPs has been carried out.[8] Guinea pig anti-MBP antisera were responsive to the somewhat more sensitive hemagglutination technique,[5,9] where titers of 300 were obtained (as compared with 300,000 for some rabbit antisera),[5] but most anti-MBP antisera have required the much more sensitive methods of radioimmunoassay (RIA) and enzyme-linked immunosorbent assay (ELISA) to capture and utilize a much diminished MBP-binding capacity. The liquid-phase type RIAs will be discussed first:

(ii)   Measurement of the antigen-binding capacity (ABC) of an anti-MBP antiserum. The molar ABC of an antiserum, i.e. the effective concentration of antibody binding sites, is readily obtained by RIA from the slope of a binding curve relating amount of radioligand bound per volume of antiserum at a given concentration of radioligand. In the example shown (Fig. 1) a variable amount of antibody (0-2 µl) was used with a constant amount of radi-oligand (7.23 pmol MBP) to produce a relatively linear binding curve (r^2 = 0.999) through the given points.[10] The slope was 0.664 pmol/µl), thus giving an ABC of 664 nM. With radiolabeled MBP, as with many other radioligands, the relatively linear portion of a typical binding curve occurs up to perhaps only 30-40 percent binding of the radioligand present; thus, it is important to make sure that even the largest quantity of antiserum used in such an assay still falls within the linear region.

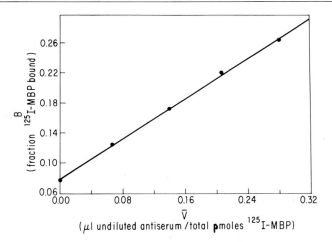

Figure 1. Typical binding curve for a multipoint variable anti-MBP antibody radioimmunoassay. The amount of ^{125}I-MBP was kept constant at 7.23 pmol and the volume of antiserum ranged in 0.5-µl amounts from 0 to 2 µl. The total volume was kept constant at 100 µl with 50% normal rabbit serum. The slope gives the antigenic binding capacity (ABC) of the antiserum, 0.664 pmol/µl or 664 nM. (From Day and Varitek.[10] Reprinted with permission from Publications of the American Society for Microbiology.)

(iii) <u>Non-specific binding</u>. A large percentage of labelled MBP, in the range of concentrations suitable for RIAs, will bind non-specifically to a number of serum components as well as to the surfaces of reaction tubes, and will remain bound as an unsuitable contaminant after immune complex separation, if steps are not taken to con-trol such binding. In the assay depicted by Figure 1 it can be seen that even at 0 µl of antiserum there is a non-

specific amount of 7.84% of labeled MBP that separates
with the immune complex. This is considered very accept-
able, with double the amount still usable for ABC determinations. The crucial factor here is to keep the non-
specific effect as constant as possible from tube to tube
for a given radioligand preparation by heeding some basic
rules:

> Keep the volume of reaction mixtures
> constant regardless of the amount of
> antiserum used from tube to tube.

> Balance the volume with normal or non-
> specific serum to keep the quantities of
> various serum components as constant as
> possible.

> After separation of the immune complex
> wash the complex as many times as neces-
> sary to remove entrained and loosely
> bound non-specific entities or dilute
> the complex several-fold just before
> separation.

The use of ^{22}Na as a volume marker in Farr-type RIAs[11,12] will
often obviate the need to wash separated immune complexes,
the amount of bound ^{22}Na being a measure of solvent remaining after the initial separation; in the case of MBP, however, the proportion of ^{22}Na remaining after the initial
separation is higher than that represented by entrained
volumes -- an indication that washing is a prerequisite to
a really successful RIA for MBP and that use of ^{22}Na does
not obviate such a step. In the RIAs of synthetic MBP
peptides representing sequences between residues 59 and 89
the non-specific effect has been noticeably less, with
radioligand binding at 0 µl of antiserum kept within the
range of 0.5 - 2.5%; moreover, ^{22}Na has been successfully
used as a solvent marker, decreasing the needed washing
steps to one.[13] It is unclear at this time whether labeled
short peptide sequences representing all other regions of
the MBP molecule will exhibit the same unobtrusive non-
specific behavior of peptides within 59-89 or whether they
will behave like MBP or worse in this regard. Labeled
peptides representing the triprolyl region, at least, were
found to bind non-specifically even less than the peptides
from 59-89.[14]

    (iv) Methods of radioiodination. The direct radioio-
dination of MBP, MBP peptides, and other myelin components
is such a central feature of most radioimmunoassay techniques that a brief overview of iodination chemistry and
its effect upon proteins and peptides is in order. The

basic reactions of iodine with proteins, as summarized 30 years ago by Hughes,[15] form the basis of all methods of radioiodination including those introduced within the last few years. The essential step would now be regarded as a transient disproportionation of the iodine molecule into positive and negative ions with the substitution of the positively charged iodinium ion for hydrogen on the rings of exposed tyrosyl, monoiodotyrosyl, and histidyl residues, and the release of a hydrogen ion (reactions 1-3, Fig. 2). The rate of reaction of iodine with the phenolic group of tyrosine is slightly faster than that with the imidazole ring of histidine, and the rate with an already formed monoiodotyrosyl group is even faster, thus favoring the formation of di-iodotyrosine. This must be kept in

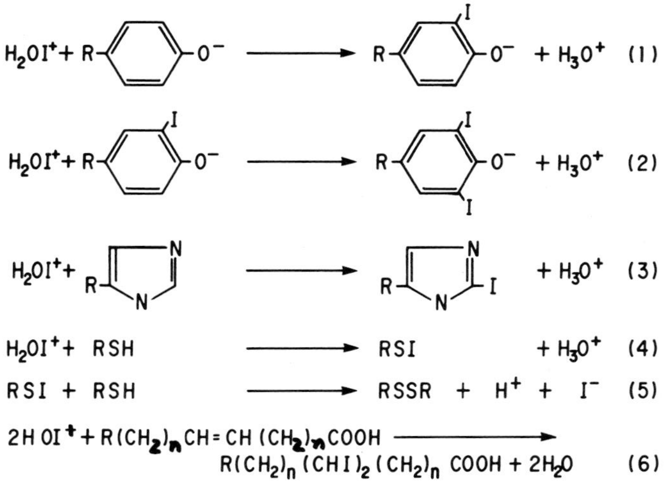

$$H_2OI^+ + R-\underset{}{\bigcirc}-O^- \longrightarrow R-\underset{}{\bigcirc}^{I}-O^- + H_3O^+ \quad (1)$$

$$H_2OI^+ + R-\underset{}{\bigcirc}^{I}-O^- \longrightarrow R-\underset{I}{\bigcirc}^{I}-O^- + H_3O^+ \quad (2)$$

$$H_2OI^+ + R-\underset{N}{\boxed{}}^{N} \longrightarrow R-\underset{N}{\boxed{}}^{N}-I + H_3O^+ \quad (3)$$

$$H_2OI^+ + RSH \longrightarrow RSI + H_3O^+ \quad (4)$$

$$RSI + RSH \longrightarrow RSSR + H^+ + I^- \quad (5)$$

$$2H\,OI^+ + R(CH_2)_n CH=CH(CH_2)_n COOH \longrightarrow$$
$$R(CH_2)_n (CHI)_2 (CH_2)_n COOH + 2H_2O \quad (6)$$

Figure 2. Reactions of iodine with some constituents of myelin membranes.

mind in the labeling of certain tyrosine-containing antigenic determinants where a monoiodotyrosyl group might still be accommodated by an antibody binding site while diiodotyrosyl might lack the required degree of complementarity. Monoiodo- and diiodopeptides can be separated by the method of reverse-phase HPLC of Seidah et al.[16] The reaction of iodine with sulfhydryl groups (reaction 4, Fig. 2) is so very much more rapid than that with even monoiodotyrosine, that available SH groups are always satisfied before any other receptive groups with the formation of a frequently unstable sulfenyl iodide (Fig. 3).

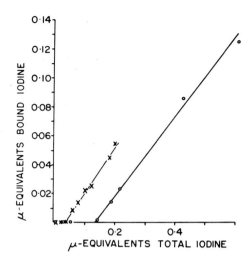

Figure 3. Uptake of iodine by two different preparations of immunoglobulins during radioiodination using the KI-NO$_2$ procedure. In the particular procedure used, 0.025 μ-equivalents would give 1 iodine atom/globulin molecule. Different amounts of iodine were consumed by trace contaminants before addition of iodine began. (From Fritz et al.[17] Reprinted with permission from Pergamon Press, Ltd.)

This is a particularly serious problem in the trace iodination of even relatively pure proteins with carrier free radioiodine since a contaminant as little as 0.1% but rich in SH groups may consume a considerable portion if not all available I$_2$. The problem can be circumvented without further purification by labeling with radioiodine in the presence of added carrier iodine (as in the KI-NO$_2$ method of Fritz et al.[17]) or pre-oxidizing the sulfhydryl groups (as in the particular chloramine-T method of Sonoda and Schlamowitz[18]).

The addition of iodine across the double bonds of unsaturated fatty acids (the chemical basis for the well-known iodine number) is not a reaction with which protein chemists would normally concern themselves, but it is (or should be) a matter of real concern to myelin researchers. Even highly purified myelin basic protein may contain a trace of lipid contamination, unsaturated fatty acid components of which will invariably form a substantial part. Thus, for example, radioiodinated MBP will invariably contain a low molecular weight portion that will, on SDS-

PAGE analysis, separate as a fast-moving radioactive band not easily detected by routine protein-staining procedures. Radioiodination of isolated proteolipid protein will also present problems unless procedures are taken either to saturate the double bonds or to separate the trace-labeled contaminants.

There are essentially two major kinds of direct iodination; hence, the methods of iodination fall into two classes also -- those in which the theoretical iodination yield is 50% because the I^- ion is not further utilized, and those in which the theoretical yield is nearly 100% because the I^- ion continues to form new I_2 which then disproportionates to additional active I^+ plus reusable I^- and so on until essentially all I^- is consumed. There is a third based on iodination with ICl[19] in which the disproportionation results theoretically into 100% usable I^+ and inactive Cl^- (but practically into 60-70% usable I^+).

The reactions approaching 100% yield are often preferred because of the economy in maximum use of radioiodine, the ones involving use of chloramineT[18,20] or lactoperoxidase[21] having the greatest popularity. Both allow for the mixing of iodide and protein prior to formation of I_2 to maximize randomness of the molecular iodination procedure. Carrier iodide can also be added[18] to increase the proportion of ligand molecules containing iodine atoms in the event that the labeled ligand competes only poorly with the remaining unlabeled molecules. Practical iodination yields are usually 70-80%. Solid phase radioiodination (Iodogenation)[22] has the advantage not only of intimate mixing of radioiodine and ligand prior to activation but also of increasing yields somewhat and shortening the time of reaction. Probably the gentlest of this first class of procedures would be the slow and controlled electrolytic oxidation of I^- to I_2 at an anode and the immediate random iodination of a swirl of protein or peptide molecules. It should be noted, however, that in all of these procedures the reagent required to oxidize I^- to I_2 is intimately present in the iodination mixture and may in certain instances have an adverse effect upon the ligand being labeled, apart from the formation of molecular iodine per se. A somewhat milder procedure from this standpoint is to utilize pre-formed molecular iodine which, however, must then be rapidly mixed with (jettisoned into) ligand to avoid an uneven distribution of iodinated molecules. One of these pre-formed I_2 procedures is the $KI-NO_2$ method that has proven very reliable in labeling MBP[7] as shown above (Fig. 1). Another method based on pre-formation I_2 involves I_2 extraction with $CHCl_3$ and subsequent mixing with ligand in an aqueous phase.[22] Although not useful with proteins that are readily and irreversibly denatured when shaken with CHCl$_3$, this method has considerable potential for major myelin proteins as well as for MBP peptides.

In those cases in which even the gentlest iodination procedure would tend to destroy immunoreactivity through chemical change (iodination of determinant-sensitive tyrosine or histidines, deaminations, etc.) coupling of ligands to pre-iodinated acyl groups such as used for Bolton-Hunter labeling[23] is often a successful alternative. This is particularly true for smaller peptides where molecular damage due to radioiodination may involve proportionately larger amounts of the available amino acid sequence.

In trace labeling with carrier-free radioiodine (usually ^{125}I) attention must be paid to the specific activity of the labeled product and the proportion of ligand molecules containing radioactive iodine atoms. For example, the labeling of 20 nmoles ligand with 2 mCi [125]I (0.92 nmole) with an efficiency of 80%, would result in an average of slightly less than 4 molecules labeled out of a hundred. Even at this low level as many as 1 out of 4 tyrosines may be diiodinated rather than monoiodinated so that the actual number of labeled ligand molecules may be less than 3%. To increase the proportion of molecules chemically labeled with iodine atoms, we must either decrease the concentration of ligand being labeled or add more iodide, usually in the form of non-radioactive carrier iodide. There are risks either way: in the one, solvent purity becomes increasingly important; in the other, an increase in the proportion of diiodo-product may occur. The ultimate decision rests on whether the tyrosine (or histidine) target is also critical to a particular determinant -- if so, then iodination may adversely affect specific antibody binding.

(v) The main parameters of specific antibody binding -- time and ligand concentration. In their critique of various methods used for the RIA of MBP, Whitaker and McFarlin[24] advocated the use of 10-fold lesser amounts of labeled MBP than employed, for example, in the original method of Day and Pitts,[25] i.e. <10 nM labeled MBP instead of 100 nM or more. They felt, quite rightly, that a greater proportion of high affinity antibodies would be detected as compared to low affinity populations, thus enhancing the specificity of reactions. They wondered also whether the higher concentration of antigen used by

Day and Pitts[25] and others, to facilitate detection of
lower affinity antibodies, might also enhance the extent
of non-specific binding. The answer to this last question
is that under the stringent controls listed above, including adequate washing, the level of non-specific binding
decreases only slightly as one decreases the total amount
of labeled MBP 10-fold.[26]

Much more sensitive to the decrease in antigen concentration is the time factor, as illustrated in Figure 4.

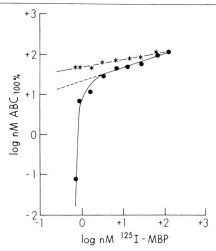

Figure 4. The effect of time and dilution upon the total
antigenic binding capacity (ABC$_{100\%}$) of an anti-MBP antiserum. The reactions at 30 min. (•) were incomplete at
the higher dilutions and required 48 hours (*) to reach
equilibrium. At equilibrium the decrease in ABC at the
higher dilutions reflects the decrease in binding of the
lower affinity populations. (From Varitek and Day.[26] Reprinted with permission from Pergamon Press, Ltd.)

At 100 nM labeled MBP there was no discernible difference
in result between 30-minute and 2-day incubation with a
typical rabbit anti-MBP antiserum, but at 10 nM there was
a decided difference, and at 1 nM the 30-minute incubation
was incomplete.[26] Within the range of MBP concentrations
shown, the 2-day incubation had reached equilibrium in
each case, and the continued decrease in ABC with decrease
in antigen used reflected the decrease in binding of the
lower affinity populations as Whitaker and McFarlin[24] had
suggested. The steeper the slope of this dual-dilution

effect the greater the proportion of lower affinity antibodies.[26] With increasing dilution of antigen, of course,
antisera must also be diluted in order to keep within the
antibody range directed by the linear portion of the binding curve -- hence, the name dual-dilution given to the
effect. The ABC at any given level of MBP, however, is
corrected for antibody dilution and written in terms of
undiluted antisera.

  (vi) <u>Separation of antibody-bound MBP for free ligand</u>.
In keeping with the original Farr-type RIAs[27] the first RIA
to measure the MBP-binding capacity of anti-MBP antisera
called for salting-out with ammonium sulfate,[28] but too
much free MBP precipitated at the concentrations of salt
needed to precipitate immunoglobulin-bound ligand to make
the method quantitatively useful. Salting-out with sodium
sulfate, however, has proven to be satisfactory.[25] As
shown by solubility curves for a number of antisera (Fig.
5) constructed according to the method of Edsall and
Wyman,[29] in which the ordinate (log S) is a measure of MBP-
bound IgG solubility and the abscissa (μ) is the ionic
strength of sodium sulfate, concentrations of sodium sulfate with an ionic strength greater than 3.6 (1.2M) would
effectively separate free from bound ligand by precipitation. For routine sodium sulfate RIAs separations and
washing procedures are carried out at an ionic strength of
3.81 (1.27M or 18% w/v). All immunoglobulins except IgE[30]
are completely precipitable at this concentration while
unbound MBP and MBP peptides are completely soluble.

  (vii) <u>A comparison of various liquid-phase RIAs</u>. Most
RIAs become identified with the procedure used for separation of free from bound radioligand even though the most
crucial steps occur during immune complex formation. The
separation procedures themselves are multiple (Table 1)
and in many ways equally effective for determining ABCs
for use in non-equilibrium competitive and non-competitive
inhibition assays; however, those requiring additional
lengthy periods of incubation for development (such as in
the double antibody technique without PEG assistance[43])
would naturally preclude their use for equilibrium-based
assays (such as affinity determinations). The double
antibody method of Fritz <u>et al</u>.,[33] the gel filtration
method of Lennon <u>et al</u>.,[34] the dextran-charcoal method of
Schmid <u>et al</u>.,[39] and the current sodium sulfate method of
Day and Varitek[10] have been particularly effective in determining the ABCs of various anti-MBP antisera.
  (viii) <u>Two-step inhibition RIAs</u>. Most of the radioimmunoassay procedures have been directed more to the

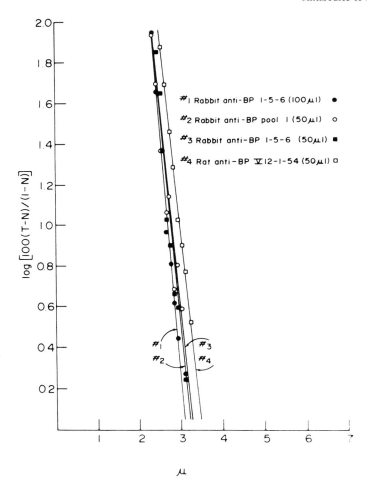

Figure 5. Salting out curves of immune complexes of antibody-bound ^{125}I-MBP in the manner of Edsall and Wyman[29] in
sodium sulfate solutions. Curves 1-3 represented different rabbit anti-MBP antisera; curve 4, a rat anti-MBP
antiserum. At an ionic strength (μ) of 3.8 or 1.27M sodium sulfate immune complexes were found to be effectively
100% precipitable; at μ<2.5 (0.84M) most complexes remained soluble. ^{125}I-MBP in the presence of 50% normal
serum remained soluble at all concentrations of sodium
sulfate except for a constant 7.5% non-specific amount at
μ>3.8. (From Day and Pitts.[25] Reprinted with permission
from Pergamon Press, Ltd.)

Table 1: Radioimmunoassays for the Measurement of Anti-MBP Antisera

Method	Formation of Immune Complex				
	Concentration of Labelled MBP in Reaction Mixture	Dilution of Antiserum in Reaction Mixture	Volume of Reaction Mixture	Protein Content of Medium, Serum (S), BSA	Time and Temperature of Incubation
Double antibody	54-76 nM	Variable	100 μl	>75% S	1 hr, 37°C
Double antibody	10 nM	1/11	110 μl	0.05% S	1 hr, 37°C
Double antibody	1 nM	1/4	400 μl	50% S	20 hr, 4°C
Double antibody	25 nM	1/40	800 μl	1% BSA	18 hr, 4°C
Double antibody	0.015 nM	Variable	1000 μl	10% S	2 hr, 37°C
Gel filtration	>500 nM	1/1.25	250 μl	80% S	12-24 hr, 4°C
Gel filtration	2.2 nM	Variable	1000 μl	10% S	24 hr, 4°C
Gel centrifugation	0.05 nM	Variable	100 μl	30% S	30 min, rm temp
Dextran-charcoal	0.001-0.13 nM	Variable	500 μl	10% S	>48 hr, 4°C
Ethanol	0.1-0.2 nM	1/100	515 μl	0.5% S	18-24 hr, 4°C
Sodium sulfate, original	10-1000 nM	Variable	300 μl	50% S	5 min, 25°C
Sodium sulfate, current	0.1-100 nM	Variable	100 μl	50% S	24-48 hr, 4°C

Separation of Bound MBP From Free					Reference
Separation Reagent	Method of Separation	Time of Incubation With Separation Reagent	Separation Time	Washes	
2nd Ab	Centrif	Unknown	Unknown	3	40
2nd Ab	Centrif	30 min, 37 C +2 hr, 4 C	150 min	None reported	31
2nd Ab	Centrif.	20 hr, 4 C	30 min	Reported	32
2nd Ab	Centrif.	18 hr, 4 C	30 min	Dilution method	33
2nd Ab	Centrif	1 hr, 37 C, +1 hr, 0 C	30 min	None	37
Seph G100	Filtrat	1 min, rm temp	Negligible	None	35
Seph G100	Filtrat	1 min, rm temp	Negligible	None	34
Silica gel	Centrif	30 min, rm temp	30 min	None	36
Dextran-charcoal	Centrif	None	10 min	Dilution method	39
Ethanol	Centrif	30 min, 4 C	40 min	None	38
Na_2SO_4	Centrif	60 min, 30 C	30 min	3	25
Na_2SO_4	Centrif	30 min, 30 C	20 min	3	10

measurement of levels of MBP, MBP fragments, and cross-reactive ligands in biological fluids than for the direct determination of antibody activity. And most of these in turn have involved the non-equilibrium two-step procedure of mixing unlabeled MBP standard solutions or unknowns with reagent antisera at some period prior to the addition of labeled ligand. The MBP standard curve in Figure 6, taken from the dextran–charcoal RIA report of Schmid et al.,[39] is typical of the result: 50% inhibition of ^{125}I–MBP binding when 200 μl of 5 nM MBP is incubated with 100 μl reagent antiserum for 48 hours in the first step followed in the second step by 200 μl ^{125}I–MBP (0.001 – 0.013 nM) for an additional 72 hours. McPherson and Catz[37] obtained 50% inhibition with 200 μl 0.5 nM MBP, using their double antibody method (Table 1), reserving 2 hours for the step-one incubation with unlabeled MBP and 2 hours for the step-two additional incubation with 0.015 nM ^{125}I–MBP. Clearly the inhibition technique does not require equilibrium conditions but only reproducible binding with a

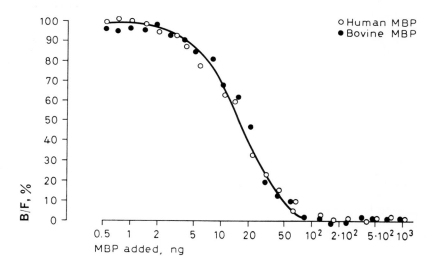

Figure 6. Standard curve for the two-step non-equilibrium competitive inhibition of human and bovine MBP with rabbit antiserum to human MBP. Percentage B/F is the ratio of bound to free ^{125}I-labeled human MBP. The ratio of antibody-bound ^{125}I–MBP to free ^{125}I–MBP without unlabeled MBP was taken as 100%. (From Schmid et al.[39] Reprinted with permission from S. Karger AG, Basel.)

given concentration of radioligand and its complementary reagent antibody. The main effort here has been to design better and better protocols directed toward increased sensitivity, the dextran-charcoal method of Delassalle et al.[41] achieving 50% inhibition with only 100 μl 0.1 nM unlabeled MBP. In their method unlabeled MBP was incubated in the cold overnight with reagent antibody (1/4500 in an incubation volume of 450 μl) followed by a 4-hour additional incubation with 140 pg labeled MBP (0.015 nM ^{125}I-MBP in terms of an incubation volume of 500 μl). Effective washing was obtained through dilution during the separation procedure. Palfreyman et al.,[42] using a double antibody technique, obtained 50% inhibition at 5 nM MBP after an overnight incubation at 4°C in a 250 μl mixture with 1/8000 anti-MBP antibody in step one; a second overnight incubation of 4°C with 0.36 nM ^{125}I-MBP in a mixture volume of 300 μl; and a third overnight incubation with the second antibody in a 300 μl final volume. With their ethanol method Cohen et al.[38] obtained 50% binding with 0.6 nM MBP after 18-24 hours at 4°C for the step-one incubation with antibody in a 500 μl volume, and a step-two incubation for 18-24 hours at 4°C with 0.1-0.3 nM ^{125}I-MBP in a 510 μl final mixture. Karlsson and Alling[43] compared the three most popular two-step techniques -- cold ethanol, dextran-charcoal, and double antibody -- using a 575 μl vol for step one incubation for 18-24 hours at 4°C, and 0.09 - 0.18 nM ^{125}I-MBP in a final 600-μl vol for step two incubation for 16-20 hours at 4°C. Then 600 μl cold ethanol (30 mins), 600 μl dextran-charcoal (5 min), or 200 μl 2nd Ab (15 min) and 200 μl polyethylene glycol (15 min) were added before centrifugation (1 hr, 10 mins, and 1 hr, respectively). It was their experience that all three techniques were comparable in many ways with a few notable exceptions, e.g. the ethanol procedure required somewhat more antiserum, and the precision and detection limit of the dextran-charcoal method was not as good. The double antibody method overall was best and "proved to be the method of choice."

(ix) One step equilibrium-competitive procedures. One has only to note the big difference in concentration between unlabeled and labeled ligands in the two-step procedure to realize that sensitivity and levels of detection of unknowns are 1-3 orders of magnitude higher than those of labeled MBP. In the one-step procedure advantage is taken of the low concentration of labeled ligand and its direct equilibrium competition with unlabeled ligand for antibody binding. Labeled and unlabeled antigens are mixed prior to addition of antibody, incubations are carried out at 4°C to near equilibrium (48 hr), and separations of free from bound antigen are made as quickly as possible. Partial displacement of labeled ligand binding is evidence of direct competition. In this technique, however, the antigenic determinants involved with antibody binding must be relatively comparable in both labeled and unlabeled entities. They need not be exactly equivalent to be useful, but the further apart they become the harder it is to quantitate. Figure 7 illustrates the point with a synthetic MBP peptide (S82) and its reaction with 4 different antisera,[44] and the dual-dilution method of assay as described for Figure 4. Two antisera can be seen to interact with ^{125}I-S82 and unlabeled S82 equally well at several different total peptide concentrations whereas two other antisera, under the same conditions and at the same

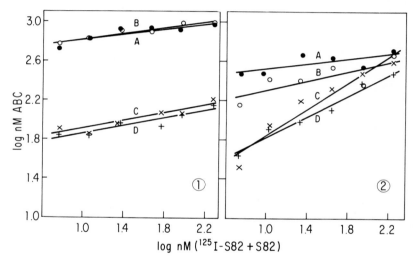

Figure 7. The effect of radioiodination of synthetic MBP peptide S82 (bovine MBP residues 65-83-Gly) on its binding with four rat anti-S82 antisera at different ligand dilutions. In both panels ^{125}I alone is shown by curves A (•) and C (X); equal parts of labeled and unlabeled ligand, by curves B (o) and D (+). In panel 1 each of the two antisera reacts equally well with labeled or unlabeled ligand. In panel 2 the top antiserum reacts slightly better with unlabeled S82 at higher dilutions, while the bottom antiserum reacts better with unlabeled S82 than with ^{125}I-S82 at higher ligand concentrations. (From Day et al.[44] Reprinted with permission from Elsevier Science Publishers B.V.)

time, react differently -- one better with unlabeled S82
than with ^{125}I-S82 at the low affinity end, the other better
with unlabeled S82 than with ^{125}I-S82 at the higher affinity
end.   Obviously, it pays to compare the behavior of labeled and unlabeled ligands with each prospective reagent
antiserum at a number of ligand concentrations before
utilizing such a system for the inhibition analysis of
unknowns.
     Inherent in the dual-dilution procedure for the equi-
librium-competitive inhibition analysis of MBP and its
fragments is the increasing sensitivity with increasing
dilution, i.e., the higher the affinity, the greater the
sensitivity.   For example, with a typical reagent anti-MBP
antiserum utilized to measure MBP activity in 25 μl normal
adult rat sera,[45] one standard deviation from baseline with
2.5 nM ^{125}I-MBP was ±74 pM; with 0.5 nM ^{125}I-MBP, ±8 pM; and
with 0.1 nM ^{125}I-MBP, 1.5 pM.

     (x) Relative affinities. Affinity is "a pivotal
element in the biological activity of the antibody molecule."[46] It follows that affinity must play an important
role in the immunopathology of reactions against self, and
that knowledge of relative affinities and degrees of affinity heterogeneity would help in the understanding of
these autoimmune processes.   To get an estimation of affinities and their range involved in MBP-anti-MBP systems,
a special method was worked out [26] based on an approach
used by Steward and Petty.[47] Since the traditional approaches used to delineate affinity constants for unitary
reactions between isolated antibody populations and single
determinants could not be used with multideterminant MBP
and polyclonal anti-MBP antisera, it was necessary to
adopt, by means of the theoretically correct Otterness
approximation,[48] a method for "the summation of the reactions between a heterogeneous antigen and a heterogeneous
antibody population."[47] The results were formulas to es-
timate relative average affinity constants (K_o) at a given
concentration of ^{125}I-MBP and to arrive at overall average
affinity heterogeneity indices (α_o) for the entire range of
concentrations studied.[26] The affinity values for one of
the two rat antisera depicted in Figure 8, for example,
ranged from about 2 x 10^9M^{-1} at the high affinity end to 1 x
10^8M^{-1} at the low; for the other antiserum, 5 x 10^{8-1} and 1.4
x 10^8M^{-1}, respectively (Table 2).

     In the recorded annals of polyclonal responses to MBP
there has been only one reported rabbit-anti-MBP antiserum
that has exhibited an unusually high ABC -- one described

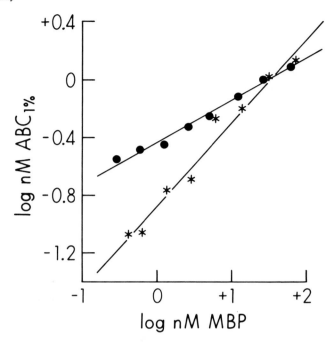

Figure 8. The effect of high affinity antibody populations on the binding of rat anti-MBP with ^{125}I-MBP as revealed through dual-dilution binding curves. The antiserum for the upper curve (•) contains antibodies ranging
in affinity from 1 x $10^8 M^{-1}$ to 2 x $10^9 M^{-1}$ whereas the other
antiserum (∗) contains antibodies ranging mainly from 1.4
x $10^8 M^{-1}$ to 5 x $10^8 M^{-1}$. When measured at 100 nM ^{125}I-MBP the
first antiserum had a lower binding capacity than the
second; at 1 nM ^{125}I-MBP it had a higher ABC compared with
the second (see Table 2). (From Varitek and Day.[26]
Reprinted with permission from Pergamon Press, Ltd.)

by Lennon et al.,[34] with an ABC of 5000 ng MBP bound/µl
serum when measured at 2.2 nM ^{125}I-MBP, i.e. an ABC of 272
µM or an equivalent of 20 mg antibody IgG/ml, an almost
myeloma amount. The average affinity of such an antibody
for MBP would be 7 x $10^4 M^{-1}$.

(xi) <u>Affinities of antibodies to individual MBP deter-
minants</u>. The evaluation of affinity constants for small
MBP peptides interacting with anti-MBP peptide antibodies
may be accomplished through conventional procedures, i.e.
by means of Scatchard and Sipsian analyses.[13,49] The form of

Table 2

Relative Affinities (K_o) and Overall Heterogeneity Indices (α_o)
for the Reaction of Two Rat Anti-MBP Antisera with Rat MBP
(as in Fig. 5) and One Rabbit Anti-MBP Antisera with Rat MBP.

Antiserum	α_o	nM ABC at different nM ^{125}I-MBP concentrations			K_o $(10^9 M^{-1})$ at different nM ^{125}I-MBP concentrations		
		1	10	100	1	10	100
Rat #4/75	0.711	370	720	1400	0.54	0.28	0.14
Rat #5/77	0.419	130	510	1920	1.51	0.40	0.10
Rabbit #E-24	0.821	490	740	1120	0.41	0.27	0.18

the Scatchard equation useful in deriving affinity constants is

$$b/f = 10^{-8} \, K \, Ab_t + 10^{-8} \, K \, b$$

where b and f are pmoles bound and free ligand, K is affinity constant expressed in conventional M^{-1} terms, and Ab_t
is the total pmoles of effective binding sites at $b/f = 0$.

Consider, for example, the Scatchard analysis of binding data for a rabbit anti-S82 antiserum in its interaction with synthetic MBP peptide S82. The amino acid sequence of S82, a copy of bovine MBP residues 65-83-Gly,
except for the Gly-His inversion at 77-78,
TTHYGSLPQKAQGHRPQDEG) embraces both a major encephalitogenic region for the rabbit (residues 65-74) as well as
the bulk of the encephalitogenic region for the Lewis rat
(residues 72-84), but by virtue of lacking Asn-84 remains
encephalitogenic only for the rabbit.[50,51] The anti-S82
antiserum was obtained from a rabbit that had temporarily
recovered from the first episode of S82-induced EAE,[51] and
it was of interest to analyze by Scatchard analysis (Fig.
9) the range and nature of the affinities involved.[13]
Variable amounts of unlabeled S82 were mixed with aliquot
trace amounts of ^{125}I-S82 and then with antisera, incubated
at 4°C for 48 hours, and developed via the sodium sulfate
technique, with ^{22}Na as a volume marker. A similar assay
was also performed with the same variable amounts of unlabeled S82 but with a constant excessive constant amount
of unlabeled YS8 (YGSLPQKAQGHRPQDENG) added with the aliquot trace amounts of ^{125}I-S82 to neutralize one of the
antibody populations. The data analysis of the unneutral

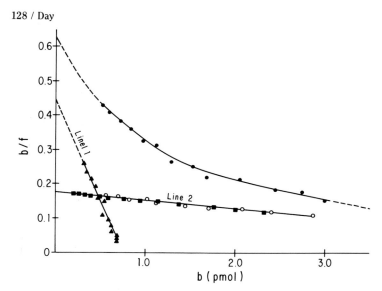

Figure 9. The experimental resolution of a Scatchard binding curve into two Scatchard lines indicating the presence of two discontinuous antibody populations (line 1, K = 5.97 x 10^{7}M^{-1}; line 2, K = 2.42 x 10^{5}M^{-1}). The data are for the binding of an anti-S82 antiserum with synthetic MBP peptide S82 (residues 65-83-Gly) in the absence of (•) and presence of (o) of synthetic MBP peptide analog YS8 (residues 68-84-Gly). Additional points on the YS8-neutralized Scatchard line 2 (■) were calculated to give data at the same f values as the unneutralized. The Rosenthal method [52] was then used to derive the points for line 1 (▲) contributing to the YS8-neutralized binding curve. (From Day et al.[13] Reprinted with permission from Elsevier Science Publishers B.V.)

ized antibidoes (Fig. 9) brought into view a curve possibly composed of two separate antibody populations each with its own discrete and separate affinity. The population still reactive with S82 in the presence of excessive YS8 had an affinity of 2.4 x 10^{5}M^{-1}. The affinity of the YS8-reactive population could be evaluated by the Rosenthal treatment of Scatchard curves[52] (an immunochemically precise method of subtracting the data points of one Scatchard curve from another at equal f values as previously used, for example, by Roholt et al.[53]) and was found to be 5.97 x 10^{7}M^{-1}. By additional inhibition analyses of the separate population it was found that the high affinity population was directed toward a tyrosyl-centered conformational determinant of the rabbit encephalitogenic portion of synthetic peptide S82 whereas the low affinity population was directed toward a C-terminal determinant of the non-encephalitogenic portion.

Most polyclonal antisera against small MBP peptides are not monospecific, that is directed only toward one determinant, but rather multispecific and usually involving more than two epitopes. And, of course, the more determinants involved the more complex is the Scatchard curve; nevertheless, it appears to happen more often than not that the affinities of the antibodies against any one MBP peptide determinant tend to be restricted and to approach affinity homogeneity. This must mean that the number of B cell clones available for response and expansion against any one MBP determinant are very limited, accounting both for the relatively low titers usually obtained with MBP immunogens and for the lack of much affinity heterogeneity of antibodies associated with a single determinant.

(xii) Heteroclitic antibodies to an encephalitogenic peptide. Heteroclitic antibodies are defined as those producing a weaker reaction with an antigen homologous to an immunogen that with a cross-reactive chemical analog.[54] The phenomenon is probably most likely to occur where there are only a limited number of clones to choose from. In any event an interesting example of heteroclisis was found among Fischer 344 rats immunized with an encephalitogenic synthetic peptide YS49 (YGSLPQKAQRPDENG). The antibodies raised to YS49 were much more reactive with an even more potent encephalitogenic peptide S49S (GSLPQKSQRSQDENG) than they were with the immunogen.[55] The phenomenon was reflected in a nearly 20-fold higher affinity of one population of antibodies for S49S than for YS49 (Fig. 10), $1.6 \times 10^{6} M^{-1}$ compared with $8.6 \times 10^{4} M^{-1}$.

(xiii) Equilibrium competitive inhibition analysis (ECIA) of heteroclitic antibodies. To illustrate the inverse ECIA pattern obtained with heteroclitic antibodies,[55] the graphic analysis of ECIA data is shown in Figure 11. The equation used for the analysis was the standard logit-log treatment

$$\text{logit } y = \log_{10}(\frac{\% \text{ max} - x}{x - \% \text{ min}}) = s \log p + s \log I_{50}$$

for which

% max was the maximum percentage of labeled ligand bound to a given amount of antiserum.

<u>% min</u> was the percentage of labeled ligand bound to the same amount of antiserum in the presence of a far excess of unlabeled homologous ligand.

<u>p</u> was the pmol ligand used.

<u>s</u> was the slope of the logit-log plot.

$\underline{I}_{50}$ was the pmol ligand needed for 50% inhibition of antibody (p at logit y = 0).

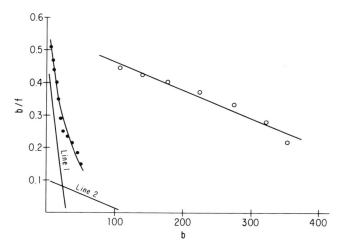

Figure 10. Demonstration that heteroclitic antibodies raised in Fischer 344 rats against synthetic peptide YS49 (YGSLPQKAQRPQDENG) react better and at a higher affinity with guinea pig synthetic peptide S49S (GSLPQKSQRSQDENG). Scatchard plot for antibody binding with S49S (•) and that for antibody binding with YS49 (o). Utilizing the method of Rosenthal[52] the curve for S49S could be resolved into two affinity populations, $K = 1.64 \times 10^{6}M^{-1}$ and $8.60 \times 10^{4}M^{-1}$. The binding with YS49 gave an affinity of $8.62 \times 10^{4}M^{-1}$. (From Day <u>et al</u>.[55] Reprinted with permission from Elsevier Science Publishers B.V.)

Ordinarily the I_{50} would be least for the homologous immunizing ligand, but in the example shown the I_{50} for the cross-reacting peptide S49S was 40-fold less than that for YS49. The difference in slope reflected the differences in affinity.

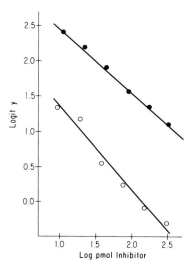

Figure 11. Further demonstration that heteroclitic antibodies raised in Fischer 344 rats against synthetic peptide YS49 react better with guinea pig synthetic peptide
S49S. Equilibrium competitive inhibition reaction with
YS49 (•) and S49S (o). Only 56% as many pmoles S49S were
needed for 50% inhibition as YS49. (From Day et al.[55]
Reprinted with permission from Elsevier Science Publishers, B.V.)

(xiv) <u>Sipsian analysis</u>. The Sips form of equilibrium
binding data[56] is useful to explore the effect of affinity
heterogeneity upon binding and to determine the heterogeneity index. For RIA data a useful form of the Sips equation is

$$\log \left[b/(Ab_t - b) \right] = a \log K_o \, a \log c$$

for which

    <u>b</u> is pmol ligand bound.

    <u>Ab</u>$_t$ is pmol antibody bind sites obtained at an
       extrapolated value of b/f = 0 in a Scatchard
       curve.

    <u>K</u>$_o$ is the average molar affinity constant (M^{-1}).

    <u>c</u> is the molar concentration of ligand used.

<u>a</u> is the heterogeneity index with affinity heterogene-
ity least at a = 1.

For the binding illustrated in Figure 12 a non-heteroclitic antiserum from a Fischer 344 rat, immunized with
encephalitogenic peptide S49, reacted equally well with
both YS49 and S49S ligands (K_o = 6 x $10^5 M^{-1}$) and was mildly
and equally heterogeneous with respect to affinity (a =
0.83) for both ligands.

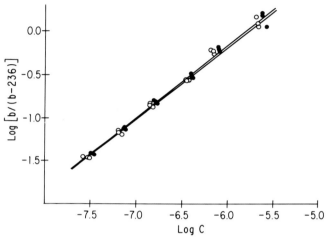

Figure 12. Demonstration that non-heteroclitic antibodies
raised in Fischer 344 rat #4 against synthetic peptide S49
(GSLPQKAQRPQDENG) react equally well with YS49 and guinea
pig S49S. Sips plots for binding with YS49 (•) and with
S49S (o). Affinities K_o were, respectively, 6.26 x 10^5 and
6.01 x $10^5 M^{-1}$; heterogeneity constants (a) were, respectively, 0.832 and 0.827; linear correlation coefficients (r^2)
were, respectively, 0.995 and 0.994. The form of the Sips
equation used (Day <u>et al.</u>[49]) was

log [b/(Ab_t - b)] = a log K_o + a log c

(From unpublished data of E. D. Day, G. A. Hashim, and
N. T. Potter.)

Continuous affinity distributions usually result in
linear plots of Sipsian data with slopes (heterogeneity)
much less than 1.00. Discontinuous distributions, as
frequently found in anti-MBP peptide antisera, however,
may produce non-linear Sipsian curves[45] signalling that an

experimental approach such as used to generate data for
Figure 9 may be useful. Affinity purification of individual antibody populations[57,58] may be another useful approach.
In either case one must be aware of and control for additional complications such as mixtures of individually
unreactive small peptides that may mimic the behavior of
reactive larger peptides[59] or the possible presence of
mixed populations with the same average affinity and affinity heterogeneity for one determinant but not another.[58]
Attempts at estimating the number and affinity of discontinuous populations through Sipsian analysis[45] can be at
best only rough approximations of the true state of affinity distributions. Thus, the neutralization procedure and
Rosenthal treatment of Scatchard data[13] as in Figure 9
remains the best approach to analyzing discontinuous antibody affinity populations.

(xv) Solid-phase RIAs. Equally as popular and precise
a method as the two- or three-step liquid-phase RIA to
detect MBP and MBP-like peptide fragments or anti-MBP
antibodies in biological fluids is the two- or three-step
solid-phase RIA. Three typical methods will be described.
In the approach taken by Randolph et al.,[60] anti-MBP antisera were readily titrated by the following sequence: (1)
adsorption of an arbitrary and excessive amount of MBP on
glass tubes to form a stable solid phase; (2) reactions in
the tubes with a titration series of a particular anti-MBP
antiserum followed by thorough washing; (3) development of
the amount of antibody bound through application of ^{125}I-
labeled anti-Ig. The titers of various antisera can then
be compared and relative strengths assigned without knowledge of exact ABCs. Linthicum et al.[61] used polyvinyl-
chloride microtiter trays for step (1) and ^{125}I-labeled
protein A for step (3) for an equally effective RIA, particularly to measure the relative strengths of antibodies
in culture fluids leading to monoclonal antibody development. Dowse et al.[62] used a two-step procedure to measure
MBP reactive with a monoclonal antibody: (1) overnight
coating of the wells of polyvinyl chloride microtiter
plates with an excess of monoclonal antibody followed by
ovalbumin treatment and thorough washing; (2) reaction
with a dilution series of MBP for one hour at 37°C followed
by ^{125}I-MBP for overnight binding at 4°C. The I_{50} of a typical MBP standard was obtained with 100 µl of a 0.5 nM solution, thus having nearly the peak sensitivity of the
most sensitive of the liquid-phase two-step RIAs.

One of the big advantages of solid-phase techniques
for detecting MBP and anti-MBP antibodies is the ability
to utilize or to capture low affinity antibody activity.[60]

This in turn makes it possible to use much higher dilutions of antisera to achieve the same end in inhibition studies[60] and to detect the appearance of monoclonal antibodies for which binding affinities may be low. It was through the avenue of solid-phase RIAs that Fritz and his colleagues were able to measure certain antigenic determinants that were conformationally hidden in liquid-phase RIAs.[60]

(xvi) <u>Liposome precipitation and spin membrane immunoassays (SMIA)</u>. That conformation may play a major role in effecting an otherwise abortive antigen-antibody interaction at relatively high affinity was demonstrated by Boggs et al.[63] Antibodies to synthetic peptide S82 (65-83-Gly), although not reactive with labeled MBP in liquid-phase, were found to react with labeled MBP that was incorporated into lipid vesicles containing phosphatidylglycerol. An alternate to direct precipitation was the use of complement-mediated immune lysis of reconstituted lipid-MBP vesicles,[64] or, even better, by electronic spin resonance measurements in SMIAs in which the spin label, tempocholine chloride, can be sued to follow the lytic events.[64]

(xvii) <u>ELISA for MBP and anti-MBP antibodies</u>. The enzyme linked immunosorbent assay (ELISA) designed by Groome[65] can achieve 50% binding of 100 μl 0.05 nM MBP with a detection sensitivity of less than 0.02 nM and thus compares most favorably with the liquid-phase two-step RIA of Delassalle et al.[41] Since it is essentially a solid-phase method for MBP measurement it also retains the attributes of that approach in screening for potential monoclonal antibody producers among various cell culture fluids. In step one MBP-coated wells of microtiter plates are treated with 100 μl of a highly dilute anti-MBP antiserum containing various amounts of standard MBP or unknown. In step two peroxidase-labeled anti-antibody is applied to determine through peroxidase assay just how much antibody remains active. The standard curve in Figure 13, if converted to a logit-log plot of the type shown in Figure 11, would give a very sharp evaluation of I_{50} values.

(xviii) <u>Immunoblot identification of MBP</u>. As a very sensitive qualitative analysis for the presence of immunoreactive MBP and cross-reactive substances, the immunoblot technique is gaining increasing popularity. It is perhaps the most powerful technique currently available to follow developmental changes in the CNS. Typically protein mixtures are subjected to SDS slab gel electrophoresis, the separated proteins are transferred to cellulose nitrate sheets, and the transferred (blotted) proteins are treated with antibody, giving a very faithful profile of the original separation. By this method, for example, Agrawal et al.[66] were able to compare the MBP proteins of CNS and PNS origin that had cross-reactivity for each other and to relate these findings to an immunohistochemical study. Likewise, Kerlero de Rosbo et al.[67] were able to detect and compare the 5 molecular forms of MBP in 14 different vertebrate species (e.g. 17 kd only in shark; 18.5 and 36 kd in toad; 14, 17, 18.5 and 36 kd in wallaby; 18.5 and 21.5 kd in sheep; 14, 17, 18.5, and 21.5 in mouse; 17 and 18.5 kd in human). Waehneldt et al.[68] confirmed the electroimmunoblot finding[67] that only mammalian MBPs exhibited the 21.5 kd component. In their study of MBPs in 8-day-old brain myelin by the immunoblot technique Schwob et al.[69] were able to detect not only the 14, 17, 18.5, and 21.5 kd molecular forms but also a 23 kd protein not previously detected (Fig. 14). By immunoblot analysis Macklin and Weill[70] were easily able to follow the development of MBP (as well as other myelin proteins) in different CNS compartments of the chick embryo up to 7 days before hatching.

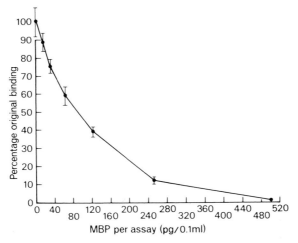

Figure 13. Standard curve for the detection of MBP by means of an ELISA. Bars show 95% confidence limits (N=9). (From Groome.[65] Reprinted with permission from Raven Press.)

(xix) Proton-n.m.r. effects and c.d. spectra. The Linthicum monoclonal antibody to human-MBP is directed toward an epitope in the 132-137 region that has the same

amino acid sequence in bovine MBP (ASKYKS) but different
in porcine MBP (APDYKP).[71] The antibody reacts with bovine
MBP but not porcine, indicating either that the serines-
133 and -137 of the bovine protein are specifically required for ligand reactivity or that the prolines-133
and -137 of the porcine protein have caused a drastic
change in local epitope conformation. The proton-n.m.r.
study of Mendz et al.[72] shows that tyrosine-135 is very
much a part of the epitope and that the prolines prevent
specific antibody disturbances of the ε-CH resonance of Y-
135 in porcine 135. Nevertheless, this local change in
epitope conformation was shown to have little effect on
the major conformation of MBP in aqueous solution, as
indicated by its c.d. spectra.

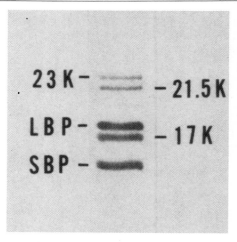

Figure 14. Identification of five MBPs in 8-day-old rat
brain myelin by the immunoblot technique. (From Schwob et
al.[69] Reprinted with permission from Raven Press.)

(c) Monoclonal and Polyclonal Antibodies to MBP Determinants.

      (i) Introduction. A very recent and up-to-date sur-
vey of monoclonal and polyclonal antibody responses to MBP
and its peptides[73] has revealed the existence of as many as
27 antigenic determinants, many of them conformational,
distributed throughout the complete topography of the MBP
molecule in at least 11 separate regions of the molecule
(Table 3 and Fig. 15). Five more have recently been
added[73a] and there are probably many, many more. It would

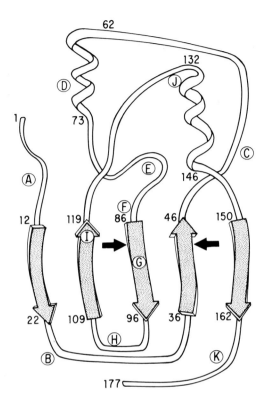

Figure 15. Model of 18.5 kd MBP secondary structure as suggested by Stoner[103] with antigenic determinant regions indicated by circled letters. Numbering made according to the revised Carnegie sequence[91] for human MBP. Black arrows indicate the Phe-Phe cleavage points. Stippled arrows indicate the β-strands forming β-sheet with a right-hand twist. Spiral ribbons are Stoner's proposed α-helices. It should be emphasized that the actual conformation(s) of MBP has not yet been established and that Stoner has only suggested the above model as one of several possibilities. (From Day and Potter.[73] Reprinted with permission from Elsevier Science Publishers B.V.)

serve little purpose here to repeat the details of that survey with its 84 references, but it would be worthwhile to consider some of the implications of the results of the survey and to raise some questions.

Table 3

Locale of Antigenic Determinants of MBP as Detected

By Monoclonal (M) and Polyclonal (P) Antisera

Determinant	Residues of MBP Implicated [a]	Region Implicated [b]	System [c]	Reference
1	1–20	A	P	74
2	15–40	B	P	74
3	1–19	A	P	75
4	20–36	B	P	75
5	1–14	A	M	76
6	1–37	B	P	77
7	88–177	H or K	P	77
8	61–87	D–F	P	78
9	79–87	D	P	74
10	65–82	D	P	51,57,79,80
11	69–82	D	P	49,81
12	80–82	E	P	82,83
13	43–67	C	P	84
14	78–87	E	M	84
15	81–90	F	M	85
16	81–90	F	M	85
17	87–95	G	M	86
18	89–99	G	M	76
19	68–87	D	P	87
20	98–100	H	P	14
21	Trp–117	I	M	76
22	Trp–117	I	P	88
23	129–136	J	M	86
24	132–137	J	M	71
25	115<det<130	J	P	89
26	115–129 or 135–155	J	P	75
27	91–118 or 161–177	I or K	P	90

[a] Numbering according to revised Carnegie sequence, Mendz et al., 1982 (91)

[b] See Fig. 12

[c] Monoclonal (M) or Polyclonal (P)

(ii)   The immunoglobulin class heterogeneity and the
multispecificity of a typical anti-MBP antiserum.   The
antibody response to MBP does not result in the emergence
of any one particular immunoglobulin class but appears to
be shared by most classes without any preference.[30]   The
classes and subclasses of monoclonal antibody immunoglobulins encountered in the survey[73] attest to this fact.
There was a time when MBP-specific IgE was thought to be
implicated in MS events,[92] but that idea was eventually
dispelled as unimportant, leaving one with the epiphenomic
conclusion that IgE would naturally be expected to share
slightly but not significantly in anti-MBP activity from
time to time.   The usual number of specificities expressed
by any one anti-MBP antiserum varies from 1 to 6 with 3 to
5 the usual number of epitopes expected.[92]   Nevertheless,
no one of the 11 segments of MBP in Figure 15 has been
found to be represented consistently, nor has any one of
the 27 determinants of Table 3 been found to be immunodominant consistently and to appear in every antiserum.
About the only consistency found in the study was that at
least 3 and perhaps 4 of the β-strands in the suggested
model failed to express B-cell determinants.   The middle
β-strand did give rise to the monoclonal antibodies studied by Sires et al.[86] and Hruby et al.[76]   The evidence,
however, was rather weak[73] for a native B-cell determinant
at the tip end of the second β-strand,[76,88] centering around
the single tryptophan residue of the guinea pig encephalitogen.   One would at first glance suspect that the complex multispecificities of anti-MBP antisera might be
considerably simplified through the use of shorter MBP
peptides as immunogens -- either native MBP fragments
obtained by enzymatic degradation or synthetic peptide
sequences of various MBP subregions.   The fact is that the
problem is not made simpler.   Immunization with short
fragments either in the free state or as conjugates with a
carrier results in multispecific antisera against a seem-
ingly expansive array of epitopes,[92,93] most of which cross-
react either poorly or not at all with antisera to the
native molecule.[92]   The cross-reactions, when they do occur, more often than not represent binding at very low
affinity and are best detected by solid-phase RIAs.[92,93]
This is not to say that the problem of multispecificity is
insoluble nor to say that it can't be solved through the
use of small MBP peptides, but only to say that it cannot
be made more simple.
     According to a group from Lerner's laboratory,[94] when
antibodies are generated to short peptide sequences of a
protein they react with the intact proteins at a high

frequency, suggesting that the immune system may have
recognized preferentially the native conformation of the
peptide; however, in the case of antibodies raised to MBP
peptide sequences, the frequency may possibly be quite
low.[73,92] There is a qualification here which injects considerable uncertainty into the conclusion[73] -- what constitutes "native" conformation remains unknown. Is it the
conformation of MBP in place in the adult on the cytoplasmic side of the myelin membrane, in a lipid environment,
inaccessible to immunologic recognition; the conformation
of MBP in the tolerogenic-sensitive neonate where the
amount of myelin produced is insufficient to contain it;
the conformation(s) of MBP degradation products present in
biological fluids during normal or disease-induced abnormal turnover of MBP; or some as yet unrecognized conformation whose topography is genetically determined and inher-
ited?

(iii) <u>Immunologic cross-reactions among MBPs of different species.</u> Martenson and Deibler,[6] using bovine MBP
as a standard and xenogenic rabbit-anti-chicken MBP as the
antibody reagent in immunodiffusion, were able to show a
high degree of identity among the precipitation lines and

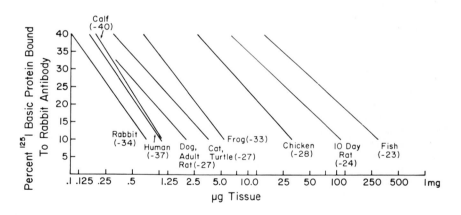

Figure 16. Demonstration that the antigenic regions of
MBP are phylogenetically conservative. Displacement of
[125]I-labeled rabbit MBP from its antibody by brain tissue of
various species. Each line was obtained from 5 points
with each point representing 8 determinations, 4 tests on
2 samples. (From Guarnieri and Cohen.[96] Reprinted with
permission from Elsevier Science Publishers, B.V.)

complete fusion in the comparison of MBPs from bovine, frog, turtle, and chicken brain or from bovine, human, rabbit, and guinea pig brain. Following the cue from Hruby et al.,[5] who had successfully used rabbit MBP as an alloantigen in the rabbit, Guarnierei and Cohen[96] used a similar rabbit-anti-rabbit MBP antiserum to show that "the antigenic region of MBP is phylogenetically conservative" (Fig. 16), not realizing at the time that the antigenic region involved was essentially the whole MBP molecule. Whitaker's cross-reaction study[8] produced probably the best evidence that antibodies can be raised to non-homologous determinants in MBP when one uses a xenogenic anti-MBP antiserum, but even there a high degree of cross-reaction was evident (Table 4). With respect to allo- and syngeneic antisera, however, would the intraspecies antibodies raised in such cases be directed primarily toward phylogenetically public or private parts of the MBP molecule? In the case of syngeneic Lewis rat antisera Lewis rat MBP,[97] it was found that greater than 80% of the antibodies in each sera were cross-reactive with a panel of MBPs from different species. Thus, the conclusion could be made that both the autoimmune and the heteroimmune B-cell responses to MBP were in large measure against phylogenetically conserved antigenic regions of the MBP molecule. When Mackay, Rose, and Carnegie[98] advanced the notion that "for thyroglobulin and BPM (MBP), genes specifying reactions to shared determinants do not seem to be eliminated by evolutionary pressures," they were severely criticized by Jemmerson and Margoliash[99] who implied that the sharing was at low affinity and not really sharing of identity but "merely cross-reactive." Since it is now known that a considerable portion of the "sharing" is at high affinity for MBP (as shown above) as well as phylogenetically conserved, it would appear that Mackay et al.[98] were correct in their notion (at least for MBP) and that Jemmerson and Margoliash[99] were not able after all to bring their immunochemical experience with the family of cytochromes c to bear upon the obviously different family of MBPs.

(iv) MBP-SF-S24. One region of MBP that one would have expected to be represented among the catalog of principal MBP determinants has remained relatively non-immunogenic, residues 65-74 represented by synthetic peptide S24.[100,101] It has all the attributes for a B cell self-determinant with a reverse turn conformation about the Gly-Ser residues 69-70,[102] a conformation that persists even when other parts of the MBP acquire an α-helical conformation when bound to ganglioside micelles. Such structures are normally immunogenic. Moreover, in one of the models of secondary structure suggested by Stoner[103] (Fig. 15)

Table 4

Cross-reactions[a] among MBPs[b]

Source of MBP	Rabbit antisera to MBP of					
	Chicken	Rabbit	Guinea pig	Cow	Human	Human
Chicken	100	9	19	53	27	33
Rabbit	4	100	97	52	73	76
Guinea pig	6	60	100	99	96	50
Cow	11	62	100	100	68	40
Human	0	83	82	70	100	100
Turtle	81	4	31	16	9	21
Rat (14 kd)	0	10	68	39	31	12
Rat (18.5 kd)	5	29	84	86	73	45
Pig	5	53	99	100	91	37
Sheep	0	62	98	100	93	54
Dog	5	38	94	98	98	67
Monkey	0	76	100	77	100	79

a/ Numbers indicate maximum percentage of complement fixed at 0.1-0.5 µg

of heterologous MBP as compared to homologous MBP.

b/ Data rearranged from Whitaker [8].

residues 65-74 are actually placed in an α-helical pattern
exposed to a hydrophilic environment. The reason for the
relatively non-immunogenic nature of 65-74, in spite of
its intrinsic potential as a good B-cell immunogen is the
presence of an endogenous and (presumably) tolerogenic
serum factor in various mammalian species that cross-
reacts at high affinity with antibodies to the region.[104]
Hence, the designation, myelin basic protein serum factor
of the S24 type. An immunochemical analysis has placed
the center of the cross-reactivity at residues 69-71 (Gly-
Ser-Leu) in the heart of the rabbit encephalitogenic

sequence.[105,105a] There is no compelling reason to believe
that MBP-SF-S24 is of MBP origin, the evidence to date
suggesting that it forms a part of an obscure non-MBP
serum protein.[104]

Fujinami and Oldstone,[106] in their study of the molecular mimicry among proteins, have very recently discovered
an amino acid sequence homology between MBP and hepatitis
B virus polymerase (HBVP) which encompasses the very same
set of amino acid residues with 68-73 (Tyr-Gly-Ser-Leu-
Pro-Gln) as the heart of the cross-reaction. Rabbit antibodies to synthetic HBVP peptide (Ile-Gly-Cys-Tyr-Gly-Ser-
Leu-Pro-Gln-Glu) were found to cross-react with MBP in an
ELISA (Fig. 17). As with MBP there is also no compelling
reason to believe that MBP-SF-S24 is of HBVP origin, but
it is clear from the evidence that the minigene responsible for a goodly portion of the sequence of the rabbit
encephalitogen is not the sole property of the MBP gene.

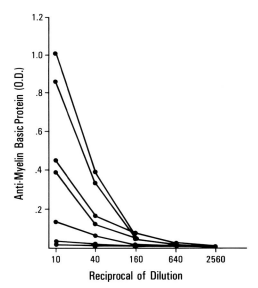

Figure 17. Antibodies to a sequence in hepatitis B virus
polymerase (IGCTGSLPQE, residues 589-598) cross react with
an MBP sequence (TTHYGSLPQK, residues 66-75), a rabbit
encephalitogenic sequence. An ELISA was used to show
binding of several rabbit antisera to MBP coated wells.
The second antibody used to develop the assay was horse-
radish peroxidase-conjugated goat antibody to rabbit Ig.
(From Fujinami and Oldstone.[106] Copyright 1985 by the AAAS
and reprinted with their permission.)

(v) <u>MBP and MBP fragments in clinical specimens</u>. The
usual procedure to search for MBP and/or MBP fragments in
the cerebrospinal fluid (CSF) and sera is through the
avenue of a two-step RIA, the comparisons being made with
the extent to which an MBP standard will bind with a reagent anti-MBP antiserum and then inhibit the binding of a
radioligand as in b-vii or b-xv. Obviously, as just
demonstrated in c-iv, it would be unsafe to assume that
just because an unknown contained specific inhibitory
activity that it could therefore be said to contain MBP or
a fragment thereof. The inhibitory substance might stem
from a non-MBP source. A moment's reflection, however,
should assure one that MBP and/or MBP fragments were actually detected by the inhibitory measures such as listed
in Table 5. Polyclonal, multispecific reagent antisera
were used in each case, a number of specific MBP determinants were involved in the total inhibitory effect, and
the likelihood of capturing entities on a non-MBP source
by such a procedure was quite small (as long as inhibitory
levels were kept above 25%). The likelihood that substances not of MBP or MBP fragment origin were involved in
the collective experiments of Table 5 becomes even smaller
since different reagent antisera were used for the different tests, thus greatly expanding the number of MBP determinants that would have to be satisfied. Thus, the group
opinion voiced in a collective report of 9 clinical inves-
tigators[113] -- that such assays would be a useful adjunct to
other evaluations "for determining recent myelin injury" -
- is certainly a safe one. Nevertheless, reliance upon a
single reagent antiserum for a given clinical study is
still somewhat hazardous and scientifically unsatisfac-
tory. In these modern days of monoclonal antibodies one
should imagine that the most satisfactory clinical approach would be for an international committee of inves-
tigators on standards to select and direct the mixing of
8-10 monoclonal antibodies, reactive with different known
segments of MBP, that could then be used internationally
for the standard inhibition RIA of MBP in clinical material. A step in this direction has been taken by Groome
<u>et al</u>.[95] Similar mixtures representing widespread deter-
minants within a desired MBP segment could be used to
search for particularly crucial metabolic fragments of
MBP. Of course, it need not be said that the use of a
single monoclonal anti-MBP antibody preparation for most
clinical investigations would be extremely hazardous.

(vi) <u>Anti-MBP antibodies in clinical specimens</u>.
Panitch <u>et al</u>.[120] discovered that the cerebrospinal fluids
of progressive MS patients often contain anti-MBP antibodies measurable by solid-phase techniques. These find-

Table 5

Some clinical investigations involving two-step liquid-phase inhibition RIAs for the detection of MBP and/or MBP fragments

Study	Separating Method	Reference
1. Radioimmunological determination of myelin basic protein (MBP) and MBP antibodies.	dextran-charcoal	39
2. Radioimmunoassay of myelin basic protein in spinal fluid: an index of active demyelination.	alcohol	107
3. Myelin encephalitogenic protein fragments in cerebrospinal fluid of persons with multiple sclerosis.	double antibody	108
4. Cerebrospinal fluid myelin basic protein and multiple sclerosis.	alcohol	109
5. Myelin basic protein in cerebrospinal fluid from children.	alcohol	110
6. Radioimmunoassay of human myelin basic protein...and its clinical application to patients with head injury.	double antibody	42
7. Components in multiple sclerosis cerebrospinal fluid that are detected by radioimmunoassay for myelin basic protein.	SDS-PAGE & gel filtration	111
8. Radioimmunoassay of serum myelin basic protein and its application to patients with cerebrovascular accident.	double antibody	112
9. Immunoreactive myelin basic protein in the cerebrospinal fluid in neurological disorders.	double antibody	113
10. Increase in myelin basic protein in CSF after brain surgery.	alcohol	114
11. Myelin basic protein in cerebrospinal fluid of patients with multiple sclerosis and other neurological diseases.	sodium sulfate	115
12. Diagnostic value of myelin basic protein in cerebrospinal fluid	alcohol	116
13. Myelin basic protein immunoreactivity in serum of neurosurgical patients	double antibody	117
14. Pre- and postoperative changes in serum myelin basic protein immunoreactivity in neurosurgical patients.	double antibody	118
15. Measurement of myelin basic protein by radioimmunoassay in closed head trauma, multiple sclerosis, and other neurological diseases.	double antibody	119
16. A double antibody radioimmunoassay for myelin basic protein in cerebrospinal fluid.	double antibody	120

ings would appear at first glance to be in direct conflict
with the results of a previous investigation by Cohen and
Gutstein[121] in which the spinal fluids of MS patients were
found to contain no detectable anti-MBP antibodies. By
the same liquid-phase RIA, Cohen and Gutstein could easily
detect anti-MBP activity in the CSFs of sheep affected
with EAE and were thus led to score their clinical results
as negative. The findings of the two groups of investiga-
tors are not in conflict, however, and the data from both
laboratories appear perfectly reasonable. As mentioned in
section b-xv, one of the big advantages of solid-phase
techniques for detecting anti-MBP antibodies is the ability to utilize or capture low affinity antibody activity;
therefore, the apparent conflict arises from the fundamen-
tal difference in sensitivity between the two types of
RIAs.[122] In continuing support of this explanation for the
apparent conflict Bernard et al.,[123] using the solid phase
RIA of Linthicum et al.,[61] were able to detect anti-MBP
antibody in extracts of MS brain; and Wajgt and Gorny,[124]
with a simple solid-phase RIA, were able to detect anti-
MBP antibodies in the CSF of MS patients. Later, Bernard
et al.[125] not only found anti-MBP antibodies in extracts
from MS brain, as in their previous report,[123] but also in
MS sera. Curiously, they could find anti-MBP activity
only in normal control sera but not in extracts from control brain. By utilizing a liquid-phase technique at its
most sensitive limits, it has been possible to detect just
above baseline anti-MBP antibodies even in the sera of
some MS patients as well as some clinically well subjects.[126] Probably the most compelling evidence for anti-
MBP antibodies in MS patients has been presented by Frick
and Stickl.[127] Using the very sensitive but highly specific
technique of antibody-dependent cell cytoxicity (ADCC)
they easily demonstrated anti-MBP antibody in the sera of
166/200 patients and in the CSF of 55/57 patients. A number of control patients also contained anti-MBP antibodies. In later work[128] antibodies to a synthetic guinea
pig encephalitogenic fragment were also demonstrated in
23/26 MS patients and 1/35 controls; thus, the existence
of anti-MBP antibodies in many humans or without MS is
well established.

(vii) Endogenous MBP-SFs and anti-MBP antibodies.
Myelin basic protein and/or its fragments may not only be
found in clinical specimens as described above in c-v but
also at considerably lower levels, and sporadically in the
sera of normal and experimental Lewis rats[129] and in normal
mice.[130] Although a considerably more sensitive equilibrium-competitive inhibition RIA was required for their
detection and measurement, nevertheless the same precau-

tions were needed to establish their MBP origin -- the use of a number of multispecific anti-MBP antisera to reduce the likelihood of detecting entities of non-MBP origin. The myelin basic protein-serum factors (MBP-SFs) appeared to be a heterogeneous collection, quite possibly small fragments of MBP, each cross-reactive with a different multi-determinant region of the parent molecule. The heterogeneity of MBP-SFs in any serum sample was defined and limited by the spectrum of binding affinities of the antibody populations represented by a given reagent anti-MBP antiserum. Some samples of normal Lewis rat serum paradoxically were found to contain high affinity MBP-SFs in coexistence with low affinity anti-MBP antibodies, other sera with the reverse pattern, and yet others with none of either antigen or antibody. Additional sera were found to contain MBP-SFs of several different affinities, but no serum sample has yet been found to contain a full spectrum of MBP-SFs. Furthermore, although some MBP-SFs were found to increase temporarily during the second week after MBP sensitization, all MBP-SFs tended to disappear in the second week and to be replaced by multispecific anti-MBP antibodies of differing affinities 3-4 weeks following sensitization.

In suckling Lewis rats, MBP-SFs are considerably more prominent,[132] their decrease with age correlating with the postnatal development of myelin, the weaning stage, and the passage into adulthood.[132] It is interesting to follow the time-course of antibody development in the adult as affected by the initial presence of MBP-SFs and to compare the results with a similar time-course in 16-day-old rats (at the time of injection) where the MBP-SF levels are so much higher (Fig. 18). Since the early portion of the time-course of anti-MBP antibody development is quite linear, it is possible to extrapolate any two time-response curves back to the point where they intersect, at the beginning of antibody synthesis. Adult curves A and B intersect at 8.32 days and at horizontal line C, coincidentally the adult MBP-SF level (expressed as negative antibody binding). Neonate curve D intersects the neonate MBP-SF level at 8.29 days, less than one hour removed from the time of origin of antibody in the adult. Measurable amounts of free antibody did not appear until the ninth day after injection, leaving one with the impression that the first amounts of antibody generated were neutralized by circulating MBP-SFs. The pronounced neutralizing effect of MBP-SFs on passively administered anti-MBP antibodies could also be demonstrated[133] with the additional discovery that the effect was cyclic and asynchronous at different affinity levels. As further experimentation

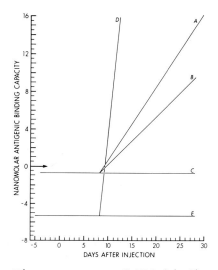

Figure 18. Time-response of MBP-binding capacity in three
different immunized groups of Lewis rats. Groups A and B
were adult; group D, 16-day-old. Lines C and E for adult
and neonatal normal rat sera showed negative binding due
to the presence of endogenous myelin basic protein serum
factors (MBP-SFs) which were at a higher concentration in
the neonate. Zero-time of antibody response was at 8.3
days after immunization, but measurable free antibody did
not appear until the 9th day after the MBP-SFs were neutralized. (From Day et al.[132] Reprinted with permission
from Pergamon Press, Ltd.)

took place the reason for the paradox -- how, in some
cases, MBP-SFs and anti-MBP antibodies could coexist in
the same serum sample,[129] and how anti-MBP antibodies at
different affinity levels could be subject to neutralization by endogenous MBP-SFs independent of each other --
became clear: The extensive affinity heterogeneity, so
characteristic of multispecific anti-MBP antisera, was not
a characteristic of affinity populations of antibodies
associated with any given MBP determinant. As discussed
in section b-xi it appears to happen more often than not
that the affinities of the antibodies against any one MBP
determinant tend to be restricted and to approach affinity
homogeneity. Consequently, an MBP fragment from one region of MBP could easily neutralize a different set of
affinity populations of antibodies from a multispecific
anti-MBP antiserum than could a fragment representative of
another region. Given that diffrent endogenous fragments

would appear in the serum in cycles different from each
other, the coexistence of an MBP-SF, bearing one set of
determinants, with anti-MBP antibodies, expressing a different set of specificities, is entirely possible. Furthermore, the neutralization by an MBP-SF would be reflected in a shift in the overall affinity heterogeneity
of the partially neutralized antiserum as compared with
the original unneutralized reagent.

(viii) Immunohistochemical use of anti-MBP. Since the
pioneering immunohistochemical study of Rauch and Raffel[134]
nearly a quarter of a century ago (myelin localization of
fluorescein-labeled anti-MBP antibodies as applied to
frozen sections of bovine spinal cord) the literature has
become rich with an extensive and varied use of the technique. In recent years attention has turned to the immunocytochemical study of oligodendrocyte function, it
having been noted by Sternberger[135] that "the absence of
oligodendrocyte reaction with anti-MBP was puzzling until
developmental studies showed that MBP could be detected in
oligodendrocytes of young rats but not of adult animals...." Through the use of a specific anti-MBP antibody, Sternberger et al.[136,137] were able to map the cytoplasmic MBP of oligodendroglia from 5-7 day old rats, to watch
how staining increased and became intense during early
myelination, and then to follow the rapid decrease in
staining of the oligodendroglial body with rapid myelination, becoming centrally almost nil as large compact myelin sheaths developed radially. Schwob et al.,[69] using
peroxidase labeled anti-MBP for their electron microscope
study of 8-day-old rat brain, were of the opinion that MBP
was definitely involved in the fusion of the cytoplasmic
faces of the oligodendrocyte processes during myelin compaction.

    The immunohistochemical localization of myelin with
anti-MBP antibodies has also found considerable value in
the study of neurologically mutant mice, particularly
myelin-deficient mutants. With such a technique Dupouey
et al.[138] were able to show that the myelin-deficient mutant
Shiverer (Shi/Shi) lacked the major dense line (MDL) of
myelin, thus punctuating the fact that MBP is essentially
trapped between the inner cytoplasmic surfaces of the unit
membrane of oligodendrocyte processes as it forms the MDL.

(ix) Adsorption of anti-MBP antibodies by isolated
myelin. In spite of the fact that MBP is confined to the
inner cytoplasmic surfaces of myelin membranes, and
should, therefore, be theoretically unexposed in undis-
rupted myelin vesicles, the protein invariably appears on

the outer vesicle surfaces of even the most carefully
isolated myelin membranes. Surface MBP of isolated myelin
membranes can be measured quantitatively by adsorption of
anti-MBP antibody,[25,139] (Fig. 19) and thus can be used as
another solid-phase alternate to soluble MBP. Since the
uniformity of the amount of surface MBP is difficult to
maintain from one preparation to the next, however, it is
quantitatively more satisfying to utilize artificial liposomes for these procedures and to incorporate known
amounts of MBP such as in Boggs et al.[64]

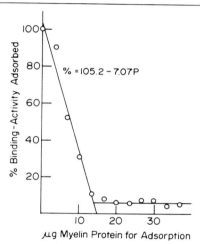

Figure 19. Quantitative adsorption analysis of rabbit
anti-MBP with suspensions of myelin. Three mg. quantities
of ^{125}I-labeled rabbit IgG in 300 µl were treated with 50 µl
suspensions of myelin, centrifuged, washed, and counted
for adsorbed radioactivity. (From Day and Pitts[25]. Reprinted with permission from Pergamon Press, Ltd.)

(x) Anti-MBP antibodies in hairy shaker disease
(HSD). Hairy shaker or Border disease is a worldwide
congenital affliction of first-born lambs originally seen
on the southern borders between England and Wales, and is
caused by a fetal virus infection that results either in
an aborted stillborn or a dysmyelinated newborn. The
lambs that do survive have anti-myelin antibodies in their
circulation[140] as measured by an in vitro technique involving purified myelin. Antibody levels appear to correlate
more with degree of demyelination than with the infective
process. Bernard et al.[125] have found that a portion (if
not all) of the anti-myelin antibodies is specific for MBP
as measured by the solid-phase technique of Linthicum et

al.[61] One does not know from these data the degree to which the anti-MBP antibodies in the suckling lambs may have reflected passive transfer from the colostrum of the mother ewes (there is no placental maternofetal transmission in the sheep[141,142]) in contrast to active synthesis by the lambs, but a steady increase in high-affinity antibody levels (as measured at 5 nM radioligand) has been noted in those lambs surviving to 22 weeks of age (Table 6). The levels are small but obviously significant. It will be important in any future studies in this area to determine the fetal age at which anti-MBP synthesis begins. Since antigens are recognized as early as 45-60 days of fetal life while some are not immunogenic until several weeks after birth at 150 days,[141] one wonders where MBP comes in this hierarchy of antigens. The answer would have obvious implications as to the stage of embryological development when an autoimmune process can become effective and when tolerance (if it exists in the sheep[143]) can be bypassed.

(d)   The evolutionary significance of MBP immunology.

Potter et al.[144] have pointed to the apparent partial degeneration of specific immune responses to MBP during evolution as explanatory of some of the unusual features of MBP immunology. One of the most puzzling has been the extreme lack of concordance among the species, in spite of their extensive sharing of MBP amino acid sequences, as to what constitutes immunologically dependent EAE, even to the constitution of the encephalitogenic determinants. The paradox is summed up by Kies,[145] "if there is some feature shared by all the [encephalitogenic] sites, it is not obvious from an examination of their sequences." What Potter et al. did was to look at the "whole" of MBP in order to assess which determinants were shared and to determine if there was some central theme.

Even though Jemmerson and Margoliash,[146] on the basis of their experiences with cytochromes c, had framed a general hypothesis that genetic specificities for self-determinants tend to become eliminated during evolution, Mackay, Rose, and Carnegie,[98] as mentioned in c-iii, pointed to certain other experimental evidence that would seem to suggest that the germ-line genes coding for the shared self-determinants of MBP (as well as thyroglobulin) did not seem to be subject to evolutionary pressures. Perhaps one could, therefore, look at the evolutionary picture to identify at least some immunological sharing among the species. Jemmerson and Margoliash[99] replied, however, that the determinants cited by Mackay et al. may have only appeared to be identical, due to cross-reactions

Table 6

The antigenic binding capacities (ABCs) of lambs afflicted
with HSD and surviving to 22 weeks, as measured by a sodium-
sulfate liquid-phase radioimmunoassay at 4.9 ± 0.2 nM ^{125}I-MBP
(Human). *

Experimental and control sera	nM ABC (range)
Normal lambs, 2-7 weeks, N=10	0.32 (-0.28 - 0.90)
Hamilton HSD lambs, 1 week, N=2	0.49 (0.03 - 0.95)
4 weeks, N=10	0.73 (0.19 - 1.54)
11 weeks, N=7	1.76 (1.02 - 1.99)
22 weeks, N=5	1.89 (1.10 - 2.83)
Baseline, 12 samplings of 1 normal serum	0.00 (-0.36 - 0.36)
Sheep-anti-MBP (sheep)	41.5
Sheep-anti-myelin (sheep)	58.4
Rabbit-anti-MBP (human)	420
Monoclonal #66, mouse-anti-MBP (human)	258

* Lim, C.-F., Bernard, C., Carnegie, P., and Day, E.D., unpublished
observations, 1982.

at low affinity and not actually shared, and that, on the basis of the evidence given, there was no reason to invoke a separate model for MBP and thyroglobulin. This argument would tend to discourage one from even considering germ-line coding of MBP self-determinants, and the recent contributions of Kieber-Emmons and Kohler[116h] to the evidence for the evolutionary elimination of cytochrome c self-determinants would certainly reinforce such a view.

There has accumulated certain other compelling evidence to indicate, however, that Mackay et al. may have been right after all, at least with respect to MBP autoimmunity:

(a)   The polyclonal B-cell response to syngeneic MBP in the Lewis rat tends to favor shared determinants with other species even when species-specific determinants are available such that over 80% of the anti-MBP reactions display shared specificities.[97]

(b)   Such a response, furthermore, results for the most part in high-affinity antibodies[26] for which the arguments presented by Jemmerson and Margoliash in their reply to Mackay et al. would not hold.

(c)   This is not to say that species-specific antibodies to MBP cannot be raised, for the cross-reaction experiments of Whitaker[8] say differently, but even in such cases the host appears to be indifferent as to the species of origin of the MBP immunogen.[92]

(d)   The recent survey of the monoclonal and polyclonal antibody responses to MBP[73] catalogs at least 27 antigenic determinants, many of them conformational and most of them shared, spread among 11 separate regions, thus bringing MBP under the umbrella of the Multideterminant-Regulatory Model of Benjamin et al.[147] Here again the selection of any particular determinant for a B cell response appears to remain indifferent as to whether it comes from a highly conserved or a variable portion of the amino acid sequence such that even the most phylogenetically conserved spatial segment of all, the triprolyl region, can be shown to be immunogenic.[14]

(e)   In spite of this rather complete inclusion of all parts of the MBP molecule as sites for an autoimmune reaction, the B cell response against any one determinant does appear to be degenerate -- best seen in the lack of any extensive affinity heterogeneity around any particular determinant,[13] in the inability of any known species to sustain an adequate secondary response against an MBP of any species,[92] and in the peculiar lack of any high affinity response near the rat encephalitogenic region of the MBP molecule.[49,49a,49b,49c]

Thus, from the above and from other scattered but extensive information on MBP immunology, it appeared to Potter et al.[144] that B cell responses to MBP had begun to degenerate even before the divergence of separate species among the vertebrates and that the continued evolutionary development of new B cell responses within any particular species has had a relatively minor impact upon MBP autoimmunity compared with continued degeneration. Presumably the gradual evolutionary loss of high affinity responses to self-determinants of MBP has involved the concomitant development of tolerance to associated helper T cell determinants within each species, with selection made against the appearance of helper T cell-induced encephalitomyelitis as a natural phenomenon. (And it must be remembered that tolerance in the sheep, for example, is different than tolerance in the rat.[143]) Other than (or because of) this necessary pairing, the mode of degeneration has been different in each species, such that the vestigial remains of imperfect pairing -- susceptibility to EAE -- has been different in each species. (It had already been postulated that high affinity antibodies in the neighborhood of potentially encephalitogenic regions would sterically hinder the binding of effector T cells and preclude the development of EAE[13,49,55].) Thus, different regions of the MBP molecule have become encephalitogenic in different species and different strains, depending on continued evolutionary changes within each species and the development of its own specific mode of tolerance. From this stance the only feature of EAE shared by most species would be an imperfect history of evolutionary development of tolerance to MBP self-determinants, different in each species, with EAE susceptibility as a manifestation of that imperfection. And the paradox essentially posed by Kies[145] in her summing up (quoted above) would be answered -- there should be no physical feature shared by all encephalitogenic sites for all species that could be gleaned by an examination of their amino acid sequences.

ANTIBODIES TO OTHER COMPONENTS OF MYELIN

(a) Proteolipid protein (PLP)

Immunological studies of PLP have been slow to develop in spite of the fact that PLP is the major protein of CNS myelin; in fact, it wasn't until 25 years after Folch and Lees[148] first described the solubility characteristics of

PLP in chloroform-methanol that a satisfactory immunological link between myelin and PLP was finally made. Agrawal
et al,.[149] after PLP purification procedures involving
solubilization in SDS and preparative SDS gel electrophoresis, were able to isolate an apoprotein that could be
used both as immunogen and antigen. The link was established immunohistochemically whereby specific PLP-absorb-
able antibodies to the purified PLP apoprotein could be
shown to localize specifically and unambiguously along the
myelin sheaths of CNA axons.[149] Later immunohistochemical
studies utilizing the same procedures[150] were able to define
the relative times of appearance of MBP and PLP in developing oligodendrocytes and mature myelin, showing among
other things that a shift in priority of synthesis from
MBP to PLP occurred in individual oligodendrocytes midway
through the myelination process. The problem during that
25 years had not been in raising antibodies but in iden-
tifying them once raised. For example, it is clear,
retrospectively,[151] that the anti-N-2 antibodies described
by Wood et al.[152] were directed against PLP, and that N-2,
lipophilin, and PLP are all one and the same substances.
This was not yet clear to everybody in 1975. Now that PLP
can be prepared without the use of detergents and rabbit
antisera easily raised against the purified material[153] it
will only be a matter of time before PLP immunochemistry
will have clarified a number of issues. At the present
time, however, PLP immunology is still rather sketchy.

The myelin PLP of the CNS is immunologically distinc-
tive, it having been shown by electroblot analysis that
there is no cross-reactivity between anti-PLP and the
proteolipids of a number of other membranes.[154] Yet there
is a high degree of cross-reactivity, for example, between
antisera to rat CNS PLP and bovine brain PLP as shown by a
liquid-phase two-step inhibition RIA[155] (Fig. 20). In the
purification of PLP[149] two molecular forms are obtained, the
major PLP and the minor, lower molecular weight DM-20.
Since the two forms display immunological cross-reactivity,[156] have comparable amino acid compositions, and have
the same N-terminal and C-terminal sequences, there is
little doubt that the two are similar with DM-20 probably
exhibiting an internal sequence deletion of about 40 amino
acids from the full PLP.[157] Moreover, both forms contain
residues 181-211 (BPS4) of bovine myelin PLP, as shown by
comparable immunoreactivities with anti-BPS4,[158] and share a
C-terminal hexapeptide (GRGTKF) in rat myelin PLP as shown
by immunoblot analysis with antibodies to the synthetic
peptide.[159] The DM-20 form appears to be missing in amphib-
ia and both forms missing in fish.[88] The two forms were

seen to develop in embryonic chick cerebellum several days
before hatching.[70]

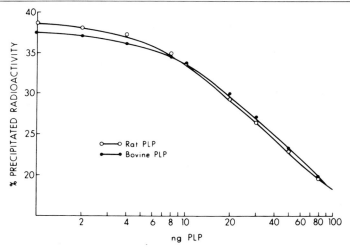

Figure 20. Cross-reactivity between rat (o) and bovine
(•) PLP as shown by a liquid-phase two-step RIA utilizing
[125]I-labeled rat myelin PLP. (From Trotter et al.[155] Reprinted with permission from Raven Press.)

     Even though there is still uncertainty as to which of
the two models, the Laursen-Samiullah-Lees[160] or the
Stoffel-Hillen-Giersiefen,[161] more closely resembles the
actual structural organization and molecular arrangement
of PLP in myelin, both roughly agree as to the placement
of BPS4 -- some of it partially exposed at the extracellular face and partially embedded in the bilayer. The
immunological data,[158] however, would seem to suggest that
regardless of the model, the determinants of the isolated
BPS4 are unrelated to any existing in situ. Anti-BPS4
antibodies did bind to the bovine apoprotein but not to
rat apoprotein, suggesting that sequence differences at
residues 188, 190, and 198 were essential to the shape of
an obvious conformational determinant (although not necessarily a part of it!). Since the immunological test to
measure cross-reactivity was based on a solid phase ELISA,
where even the lowest affinity antibodies would participate, the species difference was made the more remarkable.
It is interesting to note that antisera to the intact
bovine apoprotein were as completely cross-reactive with
the rat apoprotein in these experiments[158] as they were in
those of Trotter et al.[155] (Fig. 20). As in the immune

responses to MBP, it may also be that B-cell responses to whole PLP apoprotein single out determinants with conserved residues and conformations over those determinants with species differences.

The fact that anti-BPS4 antibodies failed to interact with myelin vesicles but did react with reconstituted PLP-containing lipid vesicles[158] suggested that the BPS4 determinants were actually near the extracellular face of myelin membranes but hindered, perhaps sterically, from reacting with antibody.

The antibodies to the C-terminal hexapeptide of PLP, however, did react with PLP _in vivo_ -- with oligodendrocyte cytoplasmic structures, but not with the major dense line of fully compacted myelin lamellae. In either PLP model[160,161] the C-terminal end penetrates the cytoplasmic side of myelin membranes and should be available for reactivity according to the Lerner dictum. That it is not suggests to the authors that the C-terminal positively charged portion of PLP must strongly interact with the opposite membrane to stabilize the myelin compact form. Other PLP determinants that also extend into the cytoplasm may not be so tightly bound since they can be detected immunocytochemically within the MDL.[162] One of the primary differences between the Lees and the Stoffel models is the orientation of the main hydrophilic loop: toward the cytoplasmic space in the one, toward the extracytosolic side in the other. Trifilieff et al.[157] hope to exploit this difference by immunohistochemical studies with an antiserum against the synthetic peptide 117-119 of PLP. Having determined that the minor molecular form, DM-20, with its approximate deletion of residues 100-140, does not interact with the antiserum (thus showing that the sequence is unique for the 100-140 region) whereas PLP is fully reactive, they are now in a position to probe the orientation question in depth.

Using a protocol developed by Driscoll et al.[78] to hyperimmunize with MBP without creating EAE, van der Veen et al.[163] were able to develop relatively high titers in rabbits against PLP. However, PLP-induced chronic progressive EAE developed in the rabbits with maximum antibody titers occurring "just prior to or shortly after disease onset." Measurements were made by means of the solid phase ELISA of Macklin and Lees[164] by which it was also determined that anti-MBP antibodies were not produced in these same animals. The authors pointed out that as a result of their experiments "an evaluation of anti-PLP

serum antibodies in multiple sclerosis patients will [now]
be required...."

(b)   Wolfgram proteins W1 and W2

        The first immunological investigation of the Wolfgram
complex of minor myelin proteins was carried out by
Nussbaum et al.,[165] only a decade ago. Of the 15-20 bands
representing the complex on polyacrylamide gels, the two
most prominent (W1, 54 kDa; W2, 62 kDa) were taken for
additional preparative SDS-PAGE purification and amino
acid analysis. Little difference in amino acid content
was found between the two or from previously published
values. Likewise, when immunological comparisons were
made by means of double immunodiffusion tests against
either anti-W1 or anti-W2 antisera (Fig. 21), no differences were found. Complete lines of identity were obtained between W1 and W2 and among Wolfgram proteins from
rat, mouse, and human myelin. Incidental to the study,
but, nevertheless, an important finding, was the discovery
that concentrations of SDS up to 0.05% can be incorporated

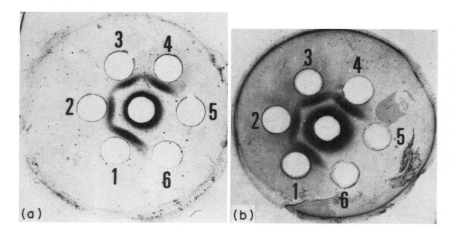

Figure 21. Double immunodiffusion of Wolfgram proteins W1
and W2 from acrylamide gel slices (after SDS-PAGE) placed
in peripheral wells. Center wells: rabbit anti-rat W1.
Peripheral wells in (a):   (1) rat W1, (2) rat W2, (3)
human W1, (4) human W2, (5) rat MBP, (6) buffer. Peripheral wells in (b):   (1) rat W1, (2) rat W2, (3) mouse W1,
(4) mouse W2, (5) mouse MBP, (6) buffer. (From Nussbaum
et al.[165] Reprinted with permission from Raven Press.)

into agar-gel immunodiffusion tests without creating unde-
sirable artifacts. From a subsequent immunohistochemical
study based on the localization of anti-W1 antibodies[166] two
previous questions about Wolfgram protein were somewhat
resolved: (1) site of synthesis -- "probably takes place
in the oligodendrocytes of the central nervous system;"
(2) origin possibly in the axolemma -- "The absence of
marking of the Purkinje cells and the neurons of the gran-
ular layer leads us to conclude that the protein W1 (and
probably protein W2) cannot be of neuronal origin."

In a combined immunochemical-immunohistochemical study
involving myelin-deficient neurological mutant mice,[167] the
technique of Nussbaum et al.,[165] was of particular value.
Equivalent amounts of myelin from brains of jimpy, quaking, MSD, and normal mice, solubilized in 0.05% SDS, were
then compared immunologically with respect to W1 content.
The actual distribution and content of W1 and W2 were
compared through the indirect immunoperoxidase technique[166]
previously used. The results showed how faithfully anti-
W1 and anti-W2 antisera could be used as myelin markers
both in vitro and in situ, the neurological mutants showing comparable W1 and W2 content on a myelin weight basis,
but showing a marked decrease of oligodendrocytes on a
whole brain equivalent basis. The observations inciden-
tally confirmed the non-neuronal origin of Wolfgram proteins. It is interesting to note that W1 and W2 are both
apparently missing in fish myelins[68] (along with PLP) and
replaced by a protein cross-reactive with P_o protein of the
PNS.[68]

(c) Myelin-associated glycoprotein (MAG)

An effective two-step double-antibody inhibition RIA
has been developed[168] to measure MAG at the level of 2-30 ng
in 200 µl total incubation mixture (Fig. 22). For the
quantitative analysis of MAG in myelin or brain tissue
samples needed to be solubilized for 5 minutes in 1% SDS
at 100°C and then diluted to 0.25% SDS (while adjusting to
0.25% Triton x 100) for final assay. The anti-MAG antiserum used for the RIA was reactive with MAG in the presence of 0.05% SDS or 1% Triton x 100 but was not reactive
with untreated myelin or brain homogenate.[169] The antiserum
originally described by Poduslo and McFarlin[168] was specifically reactive with untreated myelin or whole brain homogenate, among a group of tissues, but its true specificity
for MAG was not explored. Both antisera were raised
against a lithium 3,5-diiodosalicylate (LIS)-phenolex-
tract, but a much purer form[170] was used for raising the RIA

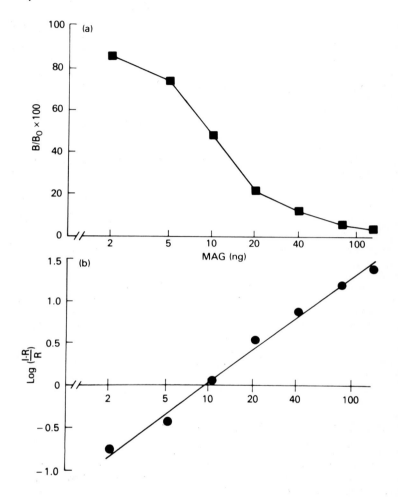

Figure 22. Standard curve used in a two-step liquid phase double-antibody RIA for the measurement of MAG. Upper panel, % ^{125}I-Bolton-Hunter-labeled MAG bound. Lower panel, logit analysis to determine point of 50% inhibition. (From Johnson et al.[168] Reprinted with permission from Raven Press.)

reagent. Thus, it is not yet clear whether specific MAG determinants have even yet been detected on the surfaces of untreated myelin (although they are undoubtedly there). The immunocytochemical use of anti-MAG antisera[171-175] usually involves enough pretreatments of tissue (e.g., fixation in OsO4 preparatory for embedding in araldite) that determinants of denatured MAG normally abound, thus making the technique useful for tracing MAG distribution. Moreover, since many of the MAG determinants are sugar moieties shared with other glycoproteins (MAG is 30% carbohydrate) rather than specific peptide sequences,[176] there is always the uncertainty whether some anti-MAG antibodies are actually MAG specific. O'Shannessy et al.[177] now recommend that mouse monoclonal antibodies reactive with MAG peptide epitopes (e.g., B11F7), or an antiserum against rat MAG, be used for detecting and tracing MAG. Mouse monoclonal antibodies reactive with MAG-CHO (such as G7C8 or F7F7) would not be useful in this regard. (It should be pointed out, also, that the recommendation for the use of anti-rat MAG should be qualified: The carbohydrate moieties of rat MAG have been found to cross-react very poorly or not at all with antibodies that are reactive with human, bovine, cat and mouse MAG-CHO; thus, anti-rat MAG antisera, even though containing, presumably, anti-CHO antibodies, could be used for detecting and tracing MAG in human, bovine, cat, or mouse brain, but not rat brain.)

Although Wajgt and Gorny,[124] through the use of their solid-phase RIA, were able to detect anti-MAG activity in the CSFs of MS patients and to observe its decrease after high-dose prednisone,[178] Nobile-Orazio et al.[179] were unable to detect levels with their liquid double antibody RIA that were significantly different (mean, 0.72%) from those in patients with other neurological diseases (mean, 0.82%), and were inclined to reject the hypothesis of a humoral response to MAG in the course of MS. However, having pointed out in our discussion of MBP how solid-phase RIAs often capture antibody activity not responsive in liquid-phase RIAs, we feel that an adequate test of the Wajgt-Gorny hypothesis has not yet been made. We also wonder, of course, what the effects of the cross-reaction of anti-MAG antibodies with other cells (such as with mouse plasma cells[180]) may have upon the levels of anti-MAG in vivo.

There is an interesting endogenous monoclonal antibody among human paraproteins that seemed at first to be specific for MAG.[181,182] Arising during demyelinating peripheral neuropathy in the human as an IgM antibody, definitely cross-reactive with MAG from the CNS as well as the PNS, the monoclonal exhibited the same immunocytochemical localization pattern[183] as a previously controversial study involving polyclonal anti-MAG antisera.[184] Whereas most studies before[171,172] and after[173,176] had seemed to place MAG immunocytochemically along periaxonal myelin fibers to the exclusion of compact myelin, the one by Webster et al.[184] held that compact myelin did contain MAG. Since it is now known that the IgM monoclonal antibody from patients with demyelinating neuropathy also reacts with a ganglioside[185] and with low molecular weight glycoproteins in peripheral nerve,[186] the study of Favilla et al.[183] can no longer be used to support the earlier study of Webster et al.[184]

At first it appeared that the human monoclonal, MAG-reactive, paraprotein was directed to a peptide determinant of MAG[176,187] since normal methods used for degradation of carbohydrates did not destroy immunoreactivity;[187] however, it was subsequently learned[188] that chemical deglycosylation would destroy immunoreactivity and that ^{125}I-concanavalin A would react with the responsible glycopeptides. The epitope clearly required the presence of the oligosaccharide moiety.

Mouse monoclonal antibodies have been developed against myelin glycoproteins with different distributions than MAG -- one reactive with CNS but not PNS myelin,[189] another cross-reactive with astrocytes[190] -- but their determinant specificities remain undisclosed at the time of this writing.

(d) Galactocerebroside or Galactosyl ceramide (Gal C).

In retrospect it can be concluded[191] that "the organ-specific antigen of brain" reported by Brandt et al.[192] over 60 years ago and confirmed by Witbsky and Steinfeld two years later[193] was actually Gal C (Fig. 23), a major glycolipid constituent of mammalian CNS myelin. Complement isofixation curves established the immunochemical identity of the natural product from the brains of 10 mammalian species with a synthetic Gal C and further demonstrated that the galactosyl head group was essential for its specificity.[194] Isofixation curves of anti-Gal C antiserum with myelin[195] (Fig. 24) then firmly associated Gal C with the myelin sheath.

Lysolecithin-solubilized myelin, in its reaction with anti-Gal C, can now be visualized not only in indirect complement-fixation reactions but also directly in immuno-diffusion reactions in agar[196] (Fig. 25). As an alternative suspensions of myelin can be used in agglutination reactions with anti-Gal C.[197] Detection of anti-Gal C anti-

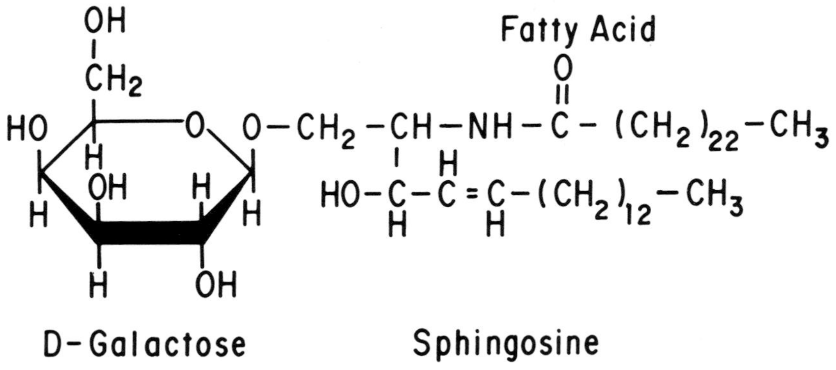

Figure 23.   Structure of a glactocerebroside (Gal C).

bodies, moreover, can now be accomplished with radioim-
munoprecipitation assays involving ^{3}H-cholesterol as
amarker in Gal C-lipsomes,[159] in Gal C-lipsome agglutination
tests,[198] and in solid-phase ELISA measurements of Gal C in
coated microtiterplates.[199]

(e) Sulfatide or Galactosyl (3-sulfate) ceramide (SF).

     Rabbit antibodies to purified SF can be raised by in-
jecting emulsions containing sulfatide, BSA (or methylated
BSA) and complete Freund's adjuvant,[200] but for testing by
microcomplement fixation must first be adsorbed with BSA
or MeBSA to remove anti-complementary anti-BSA or anti-
MeBSA antibodies.   An even better method to raise high
titer antibodies involves repeated injections of a sul-
fatide-lecithin-cholesterol-MBSA mixture.[201]   Such anti-SF
antibodies do not cross-react with Gal C or other glycolipids, but do exhibit a very weak cross-reaction with
synthetic galactosyl (6-sulfate) ceramide.   As demonstrated by an immunofluorescence test in a liquid medium,[202]
anti-SF antibodies appear to be immunoreactive with the
surface of the myelin sheath and will react with SF-
containing liposomes or myelin vesicles.[203]   The immune
damage to liposomes in the presence of complement could be
followed by the release of the trapped fluorescent marker,
4-methylumbelliferyl phosphate,[203] and was found to be dose-
dependent (Fig. 26).

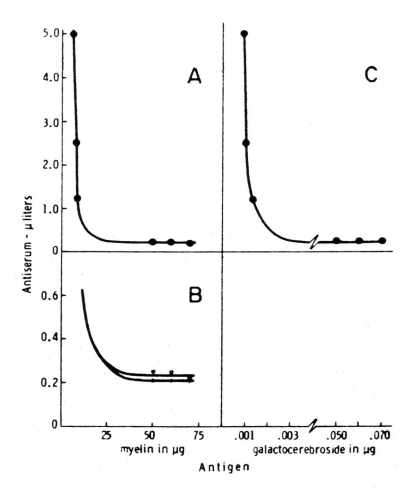

Figure 24. Complement isofixation curves of anti-Gal C with myelin (panels A and B) and with Gal C (panel C) at a sensitivity level of 3 units of complement. The analysis of Gal C was obtained through the use of auxiliary lipid (lecithin-cholesterol), now recognized as a liposome assay. (From Rapport et al.[195] Reprinted with permission from Raven Press.)

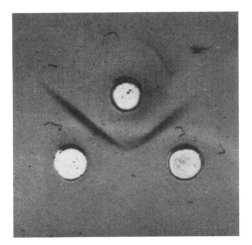

Figure 25. Double immuno-diffusion of anti-Gal C (right)
and anti-rat myelin (left) with lysolecithin-solubilized
rat myelin (top center) showing reaction of identity.
(From Gregson et al.[196] Reprinted with permission from
Blackwell Scientific Publications.)

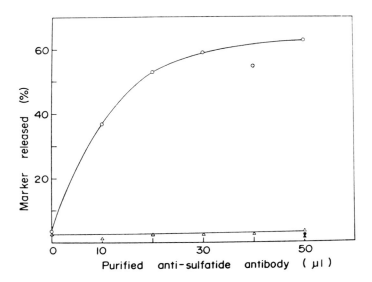

Figure 26. Immune release of trapped marker from liposomes containing sulfatide caused by purified anti-sulfatide antibody. The marker was 4-methylumbelliferyl phosphate, and its release was followed fluorometrically.
(From Uemura et al.[203] Reprinted with permission from Prof.
Taketomi and the Japanese Biochemical Society.)

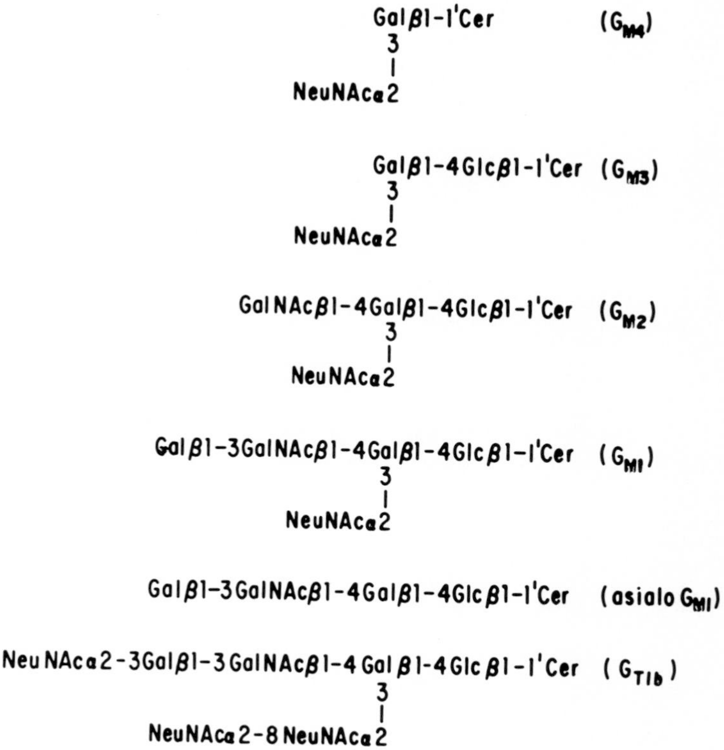

$$Gal\beta1-1'Cer \quad (G_{M4})$$
$$\underset{NeuNAc\alpha2}{\overset{3}{|}}$$

$$Gal\beta1-4Glc\beta1-1'Cer \quad (G_{M3})$$
$$\underset{NeuNAc\alpha2}{\overset{3}{|}}$$

$$GalNAc\beta1-4Gal\beta1-4Glc\beta1-1'Cer \quad (G_{M2})$$
$$\underset{NeuNAc\alpha2}{\overset{3}{|}}$$

$$Gal\beta1-3GalNAc\beta1-4Gal\beta1-4Glc\beta1-1'Cer \quad (G_{M1})$$
$$\underset{NeuNAc\alpha2}{\overset{3}{|}}$$

$$Gal\beta1-3GalNAc\beta1-4Gal\beta1-4Glc\beta1-1'Cer \quad (asialo\ G_{M1})$$

$$NeuNAc\alpha2-3Gal\beta1-3GalNAc\beta1-4Gal\beta1-4Glc\beta1-1'Cer \quad (G_{T1b})$$
$$\underset{NeuNAc\alpha2-8NeuNAc\alpha2}{\overset{3}{|}}$$

Figure 27. Some ganglioside structures.

(f) Gangliosides (Oligosaccharyl ceramides).

One of the simplest brain gangliosides (Fig. 27) and
the only known derivative in brain of a galactosyl ceramide is sialosyl Gal C (G_{M4}) (The others are derivatives of
glycosyl ceramide). Using the procedure of Ledeen and Yu[204]
to obtain highly purified G_{M4}, Jacobson et al.[205] were able
to raise specific anti-G_{M4} antisera in rabbits by immunization with a G_{M4}-MeBSA-complete Freund's adjuvant mixture.
The specificity was determined by means of a panel of
ceramides and a two-step solid-phase inhibition RIA (utilizing ^{125}I-Staphylococcal Protein A as the indicator). The
panel consisted of a number of gangliosides, Gal C, and a
synthetic dihydrogalactose ceramide of which only G_{M4} was
found to be immunoreactive (Fig. 28). Interest in G_{M4} is
high because of its specificity in the CNS of many animal

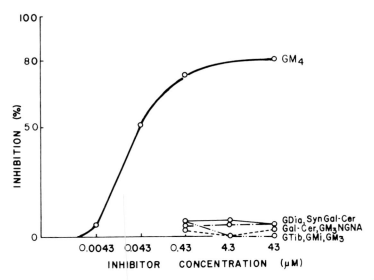

Figure 28. Competitive inhibition assay of anti-G_{M4} with various glycolipids. A two-step solid-phase RIA was used with development carried out with ^{125}I-labeled Staphylococcal protein A. Of the several glycolipids tested only G_{M4} was reactive. (From Jacobson et al.[205] Reprinted with permission from Elsevier Science Publishers B.V.)

species for myelin and oligodendroglia[206] (even though it can be found elsewhere, such as in embryonic chicken liver,[207] and can't be found in bovine or rabbit brain[208]).

G_{M1} is the major ganglioside of myelin, accounting on a molar basis for as much as 70% of the total myelin gangliosides.[206] At one time all gangliosides, including G_{M1}, were thought to be exclusively neuronal, but now are known to comprise about half a percent of the total myelin lipid.[206] Although still a monosialosyl compound, G_{M1} contains a rather complex head group (Fig. 27) from which it derives its antigenically specific pentaose nature (as well as its extensive cross-reactivity[209,210]). Although the specific orientation of G_{M1} and the other gangliosides is not yet known, it should be pointed out, in the words of Norton and Cammer,[206] that myelin is the only membrane fraction from brain that has been found to have a characteristic ganglioside pattern." Immunological disruption of that pattern may very well lead to a certain amount of myelin instability even though gangliosides comprise less than 1% of the total lipid.

Another glycolipid that is usually included among the gangliosides[206,209,211] is asialo G_{M1} (ganglio-N-tetraosylceramide) (Fig. 27) even though, by lacking a sialic acid group, it is really only a complex cerebroside. Antibodies raised against it tend to carry a relatively high specificity,[209] cross-reacting only slightly with G_{M1}; on the other hand, antibodies to G_{M1} frequently contain populations highly cross-reactive with asialo G_{M1}.[209] Originally thought to be specific for the surfaces of natural killer (NK) cells,[212] asialo G_{M1} is now known to be a brain constituent and very likely to be localized in myelin,[211] thus suggesting this glycolipid to be the common link between Thy-1 antigen and the brain. Kusonoki et al.[211] were careful to point out that their findings would not exclude asialo G_{M1} from other brain fractions, but only that it should always be listed as a myelin constituent. One wonders, therefore, whether the neuronal fraction of brain (based on an earlier study[213]) suggesting a much greater concentration of Thy-1 cross-reacting substance in neuronal fractions than in myelin) might also contain the bulk of asialo G_{M1}. Because of the extensive cross-reaction between asialo G_{M1} and antibodies to the trisialo-ganglioside G_{T1b} (rich in cortical grey matter),[210] one wonders then how much cross-reaction actually does exist between neuronal G_{T1b} and anti-Thy-1.

Gregson and Oxberry,[214] in their immunochemical investigation of the distribution of gangliosides in myelin, as compared with cerebroside, felt that the endogenous distribution of each type of glycolipid was different even though both appeared at the surface of myelin vesicles "solubilized" with lysophosphatidylcholine.

Since the levels of anti-ganglioside antibodies have been shown to be higher in the early paralytic stages of chronic relapsing EAE in the guinea pig[199] as well as in MS patients[215] (with anti-G_{M4} and anti-G_{M1} antibodies predominating in the latter study), there is continuing interest in whether such increased levels may be important to EAE and/or MS pathology. In the light of the cross-reaction study by Gregson and Hammer,[210] however, any modern pursuit of this subject should include determinations of fine specificity and affinity of such antibodies and the multiple configurational states any one glycolipid may take.

(g) Antibody-induced demyelination.

The main antigenic target of anti-myelin antisera that demyelinate mature CNS organ cultures or inhibit their formation[216,218] is galactocerebroside (Gal C).[218-224] Neither antisera to PLP,[225] MAG,[226] nor MBP[227] has been found to contain demyelinating activity. However, since there are differences between the demyelinating activities of MS and EAE sera,[227] since the demyelinating activity in MS sera possibly may be relegated only to IgG_3 among the various possible IgG isotypes,[228] and since the demyelinating activities in guinea pig anti-whole brain homogenates do not necessarily cross-react with either MBP or Gal C,[229] it cannot be concluded that Gal C is either the exclusive antigenic target or always included among the active targets for demyelinating antibodies.

(h) Antibodies to unknown cell-surface antigens specific for oligodendrocytes.

In the sera of many MS patients, as well as in some with subacute sclerosing paneacephalitis or acute disseminated encephalomyelitis, there are oligodendroglia-reactive antibodies that remain unreactive with purified myelin.[230-231] The suggestion was made that the appearance of such antibodies may indicate an immunopathologic event against oligodendroglial cells leading into subsequent demyelination;[230] however, this cause-and-effect relationship has been challenged.[232] In another report Abramsky et al.[233] indicated that the oligodendroglial-reactive antibodies would react with myelin fragments but not myelin "tissue" per se, thus qualifying the nature of the specificity. Moreover, the essential difference has been confirmed.[234] A double-antibody solid-phase RIA has now been developed,[235] using lyophilized oligodendroglia in microtiter plates, by which the difference between oligodendroglia and purified myelin can be seen to persist; however, the nature of the cross-reaction with myelin fragments remains unexplored.

Another useful antigenic marker for oligodendrocytes (other than for "dark" cells), whose chemical nature remains hidden, has been found in rabbit anti-myelin antisera that has been absorbed with kidney tissue powder.[236] After additional absorptions with isolated cerebrosides, sulfatides, basic proteins and proteolipids, and finding no WP-reactive antibodies to begin with, Roussel and Nussbaum[236] saw no essential reduction in immunoreactivity of the antisera for the specific oligodendrocytic structures. Yet absorption with purified whole myelin removed all activity. Production of this type of immunohistochemically useful antisreum was said to be relatively easy to produce.

(i) Antibodies to uncharacterized or undesignated components of myelin.

The undesignated myelin specificity of the antisera
raised by Roussel and Nussbaum[236] is apparently only one of
several determinants of whole myelin that remains uncharacterized. Another is antigen M_2 that has been found in
CNS but not PNS myelin.[237] It apparently is a protein
rather than glycolipid antigen (even though anti-M_2 antisera are capable of demyelination) and is yet not associated with any of the major myelin proteins. It may, however, have some determinants in common with PLP. Because
of the demyelinating potential of anti-M_2 antisera, Lebar
and Lees believe M_2 may possibly be an important antigen in
the induction of chronic EAE.[237]

In considering some of the earlier literature in which
the various sub-specificities of anti-myelin antibodies
could not even have been imagined at the time of publication, it is often possible now to make an educated guess
as to particular myelin structures that were no doubt
involved, in much the same way (C2d above) that Rapport[191]
in 1970 could conclude that the organ-specific brain antigen reported by Brandt et al.[192] in 1926 was probably galactosyl ceramide. In view of the disclosure of specificities of anti-myelin antibodies that are associated with
other than the known categories of myelin components,
however, it would be well to be cautious. Thus, the immunological reactions of anti-myelin antibodies with lysolecithin-solubilized myelin[238] may very well have been due
to anti-Gal C antibodies,[238] but certainly not exclusively.
One wonders, therefore, whether, in the one example of
antibody localization in vivo in myelin,[239] the antibody
specificity was directed toward one of the major antigens
such as MAG, Gal C, and PLP, or whether it involved some
other immunologically accessible but obscure surface component of the myelin sheath. Antibodies specific for
synaptosomal components and not cross-reactive with myelin
will localize in vivo in brain; however, they have short
biologic half-lives and exhibit extreme localization instability.[240] It would probably be safe to conclude, therefore, that in other examples of brain-localized antibodies[241,242] stable surface antigens of myelin were no doubt
involved. Myelin-specific antibodies were certainly present in the antisera.[243] In view of what has been written
above, however, it would be too hazardous to speculate as
to the specific myelin components responsible for the
localization.

REFERENCES

1.   Lisak, R.P., Falk, G.A., Heinze, R.G., Kies, M.W.,
     and Alvord, E.C., Jr., Dissociation of antibody
     production from disease suppression in the inhibi-
     tion of allergic encephalomyelitis by myelin basic
     protein, J. Immunol. 104, 1435-1446, 1970.
2.   Day, E.D. and Pitts, O.M., The antibody response to
     myelin basic protein (BP) in Lewis rats: the
     effect of time, dosage of BP, and dosage of Myco-
     bacterium butyricum, J. Immunol. 113, 1958-1967,
     1974.
3.   Brostoff, S.W., Immunological responses to myelin
     and myelin components, in Myelin, 2nd Edition,
     Morell, P., Ed., Plenum Press, New York, 1984,
     405-439.
4.   Webb, C., Teitelbaum, D., Arnon, R., and Sela, M.,
     In vivo and in vitro immunological cross-reactions
     between basic encephalitogen and synthetic basic
     polypeptides capable of suppressing experimental
     allergic encephalo-myelitis, Eur. J. Immunol. 3,
     279-286, 1973.
5.   Hruby, S., Alvord, E.C., and Shaw, C.M., Relation-
     ships between antibodies and experimental allergic
     encephalomyelitis. I. Production of
     hemagglutinating and gel-precipitating antibodies
     in rabbits and guinea pigs. Int. Arch. Allergy 36,
     599-611, 1969.
6.   Martenson, R.E., and Deibler, G.E., Partial charac-
     terization of basic proteins of chicken, turtle and
     frog central nervous system myelin, J. Neurochem.
     24, 79-88, 1975.
7.   Pitts, O.M., Barrows, A.A., and Day, E.D., An
     evaluation of a procedure for the isolation of
     myelin basic protein (BP), Prep. Biochem. 6,
     239-264, 1976.
8.   Whitaker, J.N., Immunochemical comparisons among
     myelin basic proteins, Comp. Biochem. Physiol. 59B,
     299-306, 1978.
9.   Swierkosz, J.E., and Swanborg, R.H., Antibody
     response to myelin basic protein: comparison
     between Lewis rats with experimental allergic
     encephalomyelitis, and tolerant rats, Immunol.
     Commun. 6, 499-515, 1977.
10. Day, E.D., and Varitek, V.A. Radioimmunoassays of
     antibodies to myelin basic protein, dual-dilution
     radioimmunoassays, and competitive binding radio-
     immunoassays to measure myelin basic protein and
     its fragments, in Manual of Clinical Immunology,

2nd Edition, Rose, N.R., and Friedman, H., Eds, Am. Soc. Microbiol., Washington, 1980, 380-385.

11. Gotschlich, E.C., A simplification of the radio-active antigen-binding test by a double label technique, J. Immunol. 107, 910-911, 1971.

12. Engel, J., and Schalch, W., Antibody binding constants from Farr test and other radioimmunoassays. A theoretical and experimental analysis, Mol. Immunol. 17, 675-680, 1980.

13. Day, E.D., Hashim, G.A., Ireland, D.J., and Potter, N.T., Polyclonal antibodies to the encephalitogenic neighborhoods of myelin basic protein: singular affinity populations neutralized by specific synthetic peptide probes, J. Neuroimmunol. 13, 143-158, 1986.

14. Potter, N.T., Hashim, G.A., and Day, E.D., Identification of an antigenic determinant within the phylogenetically conserved triprolyl region of myelin basic protein, J. Immunol. 136, 516-520, 1986.

15. Hughes, W.L., The chemistry of iodination, Ann. N.Y. Acad. Sci. 70, 3-18, 1957.

16. Seidah, N.G., Dennis, M., Corvol, P., Rochemont, J., and Chretien, M., A rapid high-performance liquid chromatography purification method of iodinated polypeptide hormones, Anal. Biochem. 109, 185-191, 1980.

17. Fritz, R.B., Lassiter, S., and Day, E.D., The effect of iodination on antifibrinogen antibodies with respect to precipitating and adsorption activities, Immunochem. 4, 283-293, 1967.

18. Sonoda, S., and Schlamowitz, M., Localization of iodine in trace-labeled immunoglobulin G, Immunochem. 8, 981-985, 1971.

19. Contreras, M.A., Bale, W.F., and Spar, I.L., Iodine monochloride (I Cl) iodination techniques, Meth. Enzymology 92, 277-292, 1983.

20. Linde, S., Hansen, B., and Lernmark, Å, Preparation of stable radioiodinated polypeptide hormones and proteins using polyacrylamide gel electrophoresis, Meth. Enzymology 92, 309-335, 1983.

21. Nerenberg, S.T., and Prasad, R., Development and clinical application of radioimmunoassay techniques for measuring low levels of immunoglobulin classes G, A, M, D, and E in cerebrospinal and other body fluids, Meth. Enzymology 73, 666-691, 1981.

22. Fraker, P.J., and Speck, J.C., Jr., Protein and cell membrane iodinations with a sparingly soluble chloramide, 1,3,4,6,-tetrachloro-3,6-diphenylglyco-

uril, Biochem. Biophys. Res. Commun. 80, 849-857, 1978.

23. Langone, J.J., Radioiodination by use of the Bolton-Hunter and related reagents, Meth. Enzymology 73, 112-127, 1981.

24. Whitaker, J.N., and McFarlin, D.E., A comparison of immunochemical methods for the detection of antibodies to myelin encephalitogenic protein, Brain Res. 129, 121-128, 1977.

25. Day, E.D., and Pitts, O.M., Radioimmunoassay of myelin basic protein in sodium sulfate, Immunchem. 11, 651-659, 1974.

26. Varitek, V.A., and Day, E.D., Relative affinity of antiserum for myelin basic protein (MBP) and degree of affinity heterogeneity, Mol. Immunol. 16, 163-172, 1979.

27. Farr, R.S., Ammonium sulfate precipitation of soluble antigen-antibody complexes, Meth. Immunol. Immunochem. 3, 66-73, 1971.

28. Kibler, R.F., and Barnes, A.E., Antibodies studies in rabbit encephalomyelitis induced by a water-soluble protein fraction of rabbit cord, J. Exp. Med. 116, 807-825, 1962.

29. Edsall, J.T., and Wyman, J., Biophysical Chemistry Vol. 1, Academic Press, New York, 1958, p. 276.

30. Day, E.D., Roche, J.K., and Varitek, V.A., Immunoglobulin class heterogeneity in the antibody response to syngeneic myelin basic protein (BP) in Lewis rats, Immunochem. 14, 31-36, 1977.

31. McFarlin, D.E., Hsu, S.C.L., Slemenda, S.B., Chou, F.C.H., and Kibler, R.F., The immune response against myelin basic protein in two strains of rat with different genetic capacity to develop experimental allergic encephalomyelitis. J. Exp. Med. 141, 72-81, 1975.

32. Bashir, R.M., and Whitaker, J.M., Molecular features of immunoreactive myelin basic protein in cerebrospinal fluid of persons with multiple sclerosis, Ann. Neurol. 7, 50-57, 1980.

33. Fritz, R.B., Chou, C.H.J., Randolph, D.H., Desjardins, A.E., and Kibler, R.F., Specificity of antisera from Lewis rats immunized with encephalitogenic fragment 43-88 of guinea pig myelin basic protein, J. Immunol. 121, 1865-1869, 1978.

34. Lennon, V.A., Whittingham, S., Carnegie, P.R., McPherson, T.A., and Mackay, I.R., Detection of antibodies to the basic protein of human myelin by radioimmunoassay and immunofluorescence, J. Immunol. 107, 56-62, 1971.

35.   McPherson, T.A., and Carnegie, P.R., Radioimmuno-
        assay with gel filtration for detecting antibody to
        basic proteins of myelin, J. Lab. Clin. Med. 72,
        824-831, 1968.
36.   Hsiung, H.M., Wu, J., and McPherson, T.A., Silica
        gel radioimmunoassay for myelin basic proteins,
        Clin. Biochem. 11, 54-56, 1978.
37.   McPherson, T.A., and Catz, I., A double antibody
        radioimmunoassay for myelin basic protein in
        cerebrospinal fluid, Clin. Biochem. 18, 297-299,
        1985.
38.   Cohen, S.R., McKhann, G.M., and Guarnieri, M., A
        radioimmunoassay for myelin basic protein and its
        use for quantitative measurements, J. Neurochem.
        25, 371-376, 1975.
39.   Schmid, G., Thomas, G., Hempel, K., and Grüninger,
        W., Radioimmunological determination of myelin
        basic protein (MBP) and MBP-antibodies, Europ.
        Neurol. 12, 173-185, 1974.
40.   Lisak, R.P., Heinze, R.G., and Kies, M.W., Rela-
        tionships between antibodies and experimental
        allergic encephalomyelitis. III. Coprecipitation
        and radioautography of ^{125}I-labeled antigen-
        antibody complexes for detection of antibodies to
        myelin basic protein, Int. Arch. Allergy Appl.
        Immunol. 37, 621-629, 1970.
41.   Delassalle, A., Jacque, C., Drouet, J., Rasui, M.,
        Legrand, J.C. and Gesselin, F., Radioimmunoassay of
        the myelin basic protein in biological fluids, con-
        ditions improving sensitivity and specificity,
        Biochimie 62, 159-165, 1980.
42.   Palfreyman, J.W., Thomas, D.G.T., and Ratcliffe,
        J.G., Radioimmunoassay of human myelin basic
        protein in tissue extract, cerebrospinal fluid and
        serum and its clinical applications to patients
        with head injury, Clin. Chem. Acta. 82, 259-270,
        1978.
43.   Karlsson, B., and Alling, C., Radioimmunoassay of
        myelin basic protein. A methodological evaluation.
        J. Immunol. Meth. 55, 51-61, 1982.
44.   Day E.D., Hashim, G.A., Varitek, V.A., Jr., and
        Paterson, P.Y., Equilibrium competitive inhibition
        analysis of synthetic peptide antigens from myelin
        basic protein as affected by the dual-dilution
        phenomenon, J. Neuroimmunol., 1, 217-226, 1981.
45.   Day, E.D., Varitek, V.A., and Paterson, P.Y., Endo-
        genous myelin basic protein-serum factors (MBP-SFs)
        in Lewis rats, J. Neurolog. Sciences 49, 1-17,
        1981.

46. Karush, F., Affinity and the immune response, Ann.
     N.Y. Acad. Sci. 169, 56-64, 1970.
47. Steward, M.W., and Petty, R.E., The use of ammonium
     sulfate globulin precipitation for determination of
     affinity of antiprotein antibodies in mouse serum.
     Immunol. 22, 747-756, 1972.
48. Otterness, I., Derivation of the Steward-Petty ap-
     proximation, In Varitek and Day[26], Mol. Immunol. 16,
     171, 1979.
49. Day, E.D., Hashim, G.A., Potter, N.T., and Lazarus,
     K.J., Immunochemical analysis of Lewis rat antisera
     to the synthetic encephalitogenic peptide S49,
     Neurochem. Res. 10, 1587-1603, 1985.
49a. Day, E.D., Hashim, G.A., and Ireland, D.J., The
     polyclonal antibody responses of Lewis rats to the
     synthetic encephalitogenic neuropeptide S55S (resi-
     dues 72-84 of guinea pig myelin basic protein) and
     its analogs, J. Neurosci. Res. 18, 214-221, 1987.
49b. Hashim, G.A., Day, E.D., Carvalho, E., and
     Abdelaal, A., Experimental allergic en-
     cephalomyelitis (EAE): role of B cell and T cell
     epitopes in the development of EAE in Lewis rats,
     J. Neurosci. Res. 17, 375-383, 1987.
49c. Hashim, G.A., and Day, E.D., Role of antibodies in
     T cell-mediated experimental allergic en-
     cephalomyelitis, J. Neurosci. Res. 21, 1-5, 1988.
50. Hashim, G.A., Myelin basic protein: structure,
     function, and antigenic determinants, Immunol. Rev.
     39, 60-107, 1978.
51. Day, E.D., Hashim, G.A., Varitek, V.A., Jr., and
     Paterson, P.Y., Immunogenicity of synthetic
     peptides sequences S81 and S82 (residues 68-83 and
     65-83) of bovine myelin basic protein. J. Neuro-
     immunol. 1, 205-216, 1981.
52. Rosenthal, H.E., A graphic method for the deter-
     mination and presentation of binding parameters in
     a complex system, Anal. Biochem. 20, 525-532, 1967.
53. Roholt, O.A., Grossberg, A.A., Yagi, Y., and
     Pressman, D., Limited heterogeneity of antibodies.
     Resolution of hapten binding curves into linear
     components, Immunochem. 9, 961-965, 1972.
54. Mäkelä, O., Single lymph node cells producing
     heteroclitic bacteriophage antibody, J. Immunol.
     95, 378-386, 1965.
55. Day, E.D., Hashim, G.A., Ireland, D.J., and Potter,
     N.T., Heteroclitic antibodies in Fischer 344 rats
     in a synthetic encephalitogenic myelin basic pro-
     tein peptide, J. Neuroimmunol., in press, 1986.
56. Karush, F., and Karush, S.S., Equilibrium dialysis,
     Meth. Immunol. Immunochem. 3, 383-393, 1971.

57. Day, E.D., Hashim, G.A., Varitek, V.A., Jr.,
     Lazarus, K.J., and Paterson, P.Y., Affinity purifi-
     cation of an acylated and radiolabelled synthetic
     derivative of residues 75-83 of bovine myelin basic
     protein ^{125}I-S79, J. Neuroimmunol. 1, 311-324, 1981.
58. Day, E.D., and Hashim, G.A., Affinity purification
     of two populations of antibodies against format
     determinants of synthetic myelin basic protein
     peptide S82 from S82-AH- and S82-CH-Sepharose 4B
     columns, Neurochem. Res. 9, 1453-1465, 1984.
59. Day, E.D., and Hashim, G.A., Format determinants of
     synthetic myelin basic protein peptide S82 mimicked
     by a mixture of synthetic peptides S8 and S79,
     Neurochem. Res. 9, 1445-1452, 1984.
60. Randolph, D.H., Kibler, R.F., and Fritz, R.B.,
     Solid-phase radioimmunoassay for detection of
     antibodies to myelin basic protein, J. Immunol.
     Meth. 18, 215-224, 1977.
61. Linthicum, D.S., Jones, S., Horvath, L., and
     Carnegie, P.R., Detection of antibodies to myelin
     basic protein by solid-phase radioimmunoassay with
     [^{125}I]protein A, J. Neuroimmunol. 1, 17-26, 1981.
62. Dowse, C.A., Carnegie, P.R., Linthicum, D.S., and
     Bernard, C.C.A., Solid phase radioimmunoassay for
     human myelin basic protein using a monoclonal
     antibody, J. Neuroimmunol. 5, 135-144, 1983.
63. Boggs, J.M., Hashim, G.A., Day, E.D., and
     Moscarello, M.A., Lipid-induced recognition of a
     conformational determinant (residues 65-83) in
     myelin basic protein, J. Immunol. 135, 2617-2622,
     1985.
64. Boggs, J.M., Samji, N., Moscarello, M.A., Hashim,
     G.A., and Day, E.D., Immune lysis of reconstituted
     myelin basic protein -- lipid vesicles and myelin
     vesicles, J. Immunol. 130, 1687-1694, 1983.
65. Groome, N.P., Enzyme-linked immunosorbent assays
     for myelin basic protein and antibodies to myelin
     basic protein, J. Neurochem. 35, 1409-1417, 1980.
66. Agrawal, H.C., Clark, H.B., Agrawal, D., Seil,
     F.J., and Quarles, R.H., Identification of
     antibodies in anti-CNS and anti-PNS myelin sera by
     immunoblot, characterization by immuno-
     histochemistry, and their effect in tissue culture,
     Brain Res. 307, 191-200, 1984.
67. Kerlero-deRosbo, N., Carnegie, P.R., Bernard,
     C.C.A., and Linthicum, D.S., Detection of various
     forms of myelin basic protein in vertebrates by
     electroimmunoblotting, Neurochem. Res. 9,
     1359-1369, 1984.

68.   Waehneldt, T.V., Malotka, J., Karin, N.J., and
        Matthieu, J.M., Phylogenetic examination of ver-
        tebrate central nervous system myelin proteins by
        electro-immunoblotting, Neurosci. Letters 57,
        97-102, 1985.
69.   Schwob, V.S., Clark, H.B., Agrawal, D., and
        Agrawal, H.C., Electron microscopic im-
        munocytochemical localization of myelid proteolipid
        protein and myelin basic protein to oligodendro-
        cytes in rat brain during myelination, J. Neuro-
        chem. 45, 559-571, 1985.
70.   Macklin, W.B., and Weill, C.L., Appearance of
        myelin proteins during development in the chick
        central nervous system. Developmental Neurosci. 7,
        170-178, 1985.
71.   Carnegie, P.R., Dowse, C.A., and Linthicum, D.S.,
        Antigenic determinant recognized by a monoclonal
        antibody to human myelin basic protein, J. Neuro-
        immunol. 5, 125-134, 1983.
72.   Mendz, G.L., Moore, W.J., Easterbrook-Smith, and
        Linthicum, D.S., Proton-n.m.r. study of interaction
        of myelin basic protein with a monoclonal antibody,
        Biochem. J. 228, 61-68, 1985.
73.   Day, E.D., and Potter, N.T., Monoclonal and poly-
        clonal antibodies to myelin basic protein deter-
        minants, J. Neuroimmunol. 10, 289-312, 1986.
73a.   Hruby, S., Alvord, E.C., Jr.,Groome, N.P., Dawkes,
        A., and Martenson, R.E., Monoclonal antibodies
        reactive with myelin basic protein, Mol. Immunol.
        24, 1359-1367, 1987.
74.   Whitaker, J.N., Chou, C.H.J., Chou, F.C.H., and
        Kibler, R.F., Antigenic determinants of bovine
        myelin encephalitogenic protein recognized by
        rabbit antibody to myelin encephalitogenic protein,
        J. Biol. Chem. 250, 9106-9111, 1975.
75.   Driscoll, B.F., and Kies, M.W., Antigenicity of
        myelin basic protein -- structural requirements for
        antibody induction, Fed. Proc. 36, 1298, 1977.
76.   Hruby, S., Alvord, E.C., Martenson, R.E., Deibler,
        G.E., Hickey, W.F., and Gonatas, N.K., Sites in
        myelin basic protein that react with monoclonal
        antibodies, J. Neurochem. 44, 637-650, 1985.
77.   Fritz, R.B., Chou, C.H.J., and McFarlin, D.E.,
        Induction of experimental allergic encehalomyelitis
        in PL/J and (SJL/JxPL/J)F$_1$ mice by myelin basic
        protein and its peptides: localization of a second
        encephalitogenic determinant, J. Immunol. 130,
        191-194, 1983.
78.   Driscoll, B.F., Kramer, A.J., and Kies, M.W.,
        Myelin basic protein: location of multiple in-

dependent antigenic regions, Science 184, 73-75, 1974.

79. Day, E.D., Hashim, G.A., Varitek, V.A., Jr., Lazarus, K.J.,and Paterson, P.Y., Synthetic peptides from region 65-84 of bovine myelin basic protein: radioimmunoassays and equilibrium competitive inhibition studies with antibodies prepared against myelin basic protein, Neurochem. Res. 6, 913-929, 1981.

80. Day, E.D., Hashim, G.A., Varitek, V.A., Jr., and Paterson, P.Y., Equilibrium and non-equilibrium competitive inhibitions of antipeptide antibody binding of parent myelin basic protein and 18 related peptide sequences, Neurochem. Res. 6, 577-593, 1981.

81. Day, E.D., Hashim, G.A., Lazarus, K.J., and Paterson, P.Y., A serum factor cross-reactive with antibodies to a determinant of rabbit encephalitogenic sequence 65-74 of myelin basic protein, Neurochem. Res. 10, 411-426, 1985.

82. Whitaker, J.N., The antigenic reactivity of small fragments derived from human myelin basic protein peptide 43-88, J. Immunol. 129, 2729-2733, 1982.

83. Whitaker, J.N., The appearance of a new antigenic determinant during the degradation of myelin basic protein, J. Neuroimmunol. 2, 201-207, 1982.

84. Fritz, R.B., and C.H.J. Chou, Epitopes of peptide 43-88 of guinea pig myelin basic protein: localization with monoclonal antibodies, J. Immunol. 130, 2180-2182, 1983.

85. Groome, N.P., Hartland, J.C., and Dawkes, A., Preparation and proportions of monoclonal antibodies to MBP and its peptides, Neurochem. Interntl. 7, 309-318, 1985.

86. Sires, L.R., Hruby, S., Alvord, E.C., Jr., Hellstrom, I., Hellstrom, K.E., Kies, M.W., Martenson, R., Deibler, G.E., Beckman, E.D., and Casnellie, J.E., Species restrictions of a monoclonal antibody reaction with residues 130 to 137 in encephalitogenic myelin basic protein, Science 214, 87-88, 1981.

87. Kibler, R.F., Fritz, R.B., Chou, F.C.H., Chou, C.H.J., Peacocke, N.Y., Brown, N.M., and McFarlin, D.E., Immune response of Lewis rats to peptide Cl (residues 68-88) of guinea pig and rat myelin basic protein, J. Exp. Med. 146, 1323-1333, 1977.

88. Hung, T.C., and Rauch, H.C., Antibody response to synthetic encephalitogenic peptides, Mol. Immunol. 17, 527-531, 1980.

89. Whitaker, J.N., Chou, C.H.J., Chou, F.C.H., and Kibler, R.F., Molecular internalization of a region of myelin basic protein, J. Exp. Med. 146, 317-331, 1977.

90. Pettinelli, C.B., Fritz, R.B., Chou, C.H.J., and McFarlin, D., Encephalitogenic activity of guinea pig myelin basic protein in the SJL mouse, J. Immunol. 129, 1209-1211, 1982.

91. Mendz, G.L., Moore, W.J., and Carnegie, P.R., NMR studies of myelin basic protein. VI. Proton spectra in aqueous solution of proteins from mammalian and avian species, Aust. J. Chem. 35, 1979-2006, 1982.

92. Day, E.D., Myelin basic protein, Contemp. Topics Mol. Immunol. 8, 1-39, 1981.

93. Price, J.O., Whitaker, J.N., Vasu, R.I., and Metzger, D.W., Multiple epitopes in a dodecapeptide of myelin basic protein determined by monoclonal antibodies, J. Immunol. 136, 2426-2431, 1986.

94. Niman, H.L., Houghten, R.A., Walker, L.E., Reisfeld, R.A., Wilson, T.A., Hogle, J.N., and Lerner, R.A., Generation of protein-reactive antibodies by short peptides is an event of high frequency: implications for the structural basis of immune recognition, Proc. Natl. Acad. Sci. 80, 4949-4953, 1983.

95. Groome, N.P., Dawkes, A., Gales, M., Hruby, S., and Alvord, E.C., Jr., Region-specific immunoassays for human myelin basic protein, J. Neuroimmunol. 12, 253-264, 1986.

96. Guarnieri, M., and Cohen, S.R., The antigenic region of the myelin basic protein is phylogenet-ically conservative, Brain Res. 100, 226-230, 1975.

97. Pitts, O.M., Varitek, V.A., and Day, E.D., The extensive cross-reaction of several syngeneic rat-anti-BP antiserums with myelin basic proteins (BP) of other species, Immunochem. 13, 307-312, 1976.

98. Mackay, I.R., Rose, N.R, and Carnegie, P.R., Germ-line detection of genes coding for self-deter-minanta, Nature, 288, 302, 1980.

99. Jemmerson, R., and Margoliash, E., Jemmerson and Margoliash reply, Nature 288, 302-303, 1980.

100. Lazarus, K.J., Hashim, G.A., Varitek, V.A., Jr., Paterson, P.Y., and Day, E.D. A rabbit B cell determinant for a conserved portion of myelin basic protein, rabbit encephalitogenic sequence 65-74, J. Immunol. 131, 275-281, 1983.

101. Potter, N.T., Hashim, G.A., and Day, E.D., Immunochemical specificity of antisera raised

against the synthetic encephalitogenic peptide SH624, residues 59-74 of the myelin basic protein, Neurochem. Res. In Press, 1986.

102.   Mendz, G.L., and Moore, W.J., NMR studies of myelin basic protein. X. Conformation of a determinant encephalitogenic in the rabbit, Biochem. Biophys. Acta 748, 176-183, 1983.

103.   Stoner, G.L., Predicted folding of ß-structure in myelin basic protein, J. Neurochem. 43, 433-447, 1984.

104.   Day, E.D., Hashim, G.A., Lazarus, K.J., and Paterson, P.Y., A serum factor cross-reactive with antibodies to a determinant of rabbit encephalitogenic sequence 65-74 of myelin basic protein, Neurochem. Res. 10, 411-426, 1985.

105.   Potter, N.T., Hashim, G.A., and Day, E.D., An immunochemical analysis of a myelin basic protein serum factor: cross-reactivity with residues 69-71 of the rabbit encephalitogenic sequence 65-74 of myelin basic protein, J. Neuroscience Res. 15, 457-466, 1986.

105a.   Tyrey, S.J., Hashim, G.A., Potter, N.T., and Day, E.D., A major epitope of synthetic rabbit encephalitogen S24 disclosed through the use of a tritiated pedtide probe, J. Neuroscience Res. 18, 493-496, 1987.

106.   Fujinami, R.S., and Oldstone, M.B.A., Amino acid homology between the encephalitogenic site of myelin basic protein and virus: mechanism for autoimmunity, Science 230, 1043-1045, 1985.

107.   Cohen, S.R., Herndon, R.M., and McKhann, G.M., Radioimmunoassay of myelin basic protein in spinal fluid: an index of active demyelination, New Eng. J. Med. 295, 1455-1457, 1976.

108.   Whitaker, J.N., Myelin encephalitogenic protein fragments in cerebrospinal fluid of persons with multiple sclerosis, Neurol. 27, 911-920, 1977.

109.   Cohen, S.R., Brune, M.J., Herndon, R.M., and McKhann, G.M., Cerebrospinal fluid myelin basic protein and multiple sclerosis, In Myelination and Demyelination, J. Palo, ed., Plenum Press, New York, 1978, pp. 513-519.

110.   Kohlschütter, A., Myelin basic protein in cerebrospinal fluid from children, Eur. J. Pediatr. 127, 155-161, 1978.

111.   Carson, J.H., Barbarese, E., Braun, P.E., and McPherson, T.A., Components in multiple sclerosis cerebrospinal fluid that are detected by radioimmunoassay for myelin basic protein, Proc. Natl. Acad. Sci. USA, 75, 1976-1978, 1978.

112.   Palfreyman, J.W., Johnston, R.V., Ratcliffe, J.G.,
        Thomas, D.G.T., and Forbes, C.D, Radioimmunoassay
        of serum myelin basic protein and its application
        to patients with cerebrovascular accident, Clin.
        Chim. Acta 92, 403-409, 1979.
113.   Whitaker, J.N., Lisak, R.P., Bashir, R.M., Fitch,
        O.H., Seyer, J.M., Krance, R., Lawrence, J.A.,
        Ch'ien, L.T., and O'Sullivan, P., Immunoreactive
        myelin basic protein in the cerebrospinal fluid in
        neurological disorders, Ann. Neurol. 7, 58-64,
        1980.
114.   Alling, C., Karlsson, B., and Vällfors, B.,
        Increase in myelin basic protin in CSF after brain
        surgery, J. Neurol. 223, 225-230, 1980.
115.   Biber, A., Englert, D., Dommasch, D.,and Hempel,
        K., Myelin basic protein in cerebrospinal fluid of
        patients with multiple sclerosis and other neuro-
        logical diseases. J. Neurol. 225, 231-236, 1981.
116.   Cohen, S.R., Brooks, B.R., Herndon, R.M., and
        McKhann, G.M., A diagnostic index of active
        demyelination: myelin basic protein in cerebro-
        spinal fluid, Ann. Neurol. 8, 25-31, 1980.
117.   Thomas, D.G.T., Hoyle, N.R., Seeldrayers, P.,
        Myelin basic protein immunoreactivity in serum of
        neurosurgical patients, J. Neurol. Neurosurg.
        Psychiat. 47, 173-175, 1984.
118.   Hoyle, N.R., Seeldrayers, P.A., Moussa, A.H., Paul,
        E.A., and Thomas, D.G.T., Pre- and post-operative
        changes in serum myelin basic protein immuno-
        reactivity in neurosurgical patients, J. Neurosurg.
        61, 49-52, 1984.
119.   Mukherjee, A., Vogt, R.F., and Linthicum, D.S.,
        Measurement of myelin basic protein by radio-
        immunoassay in closed head trauma, multiple
        sclerosis, and other neutrological diseases, Clin.
        Biochem. 18, 304-307, 1985.
120.   Panitch, H.S., Hooper, C.J., and Johnson, K.P., CSF
        antibody to myelin basic protein. Measurement in
        patients with multiple sclerosis and subacute
        sclerosing panecephalitis, Arch. Neurol. 37,
        206-209, 1980.
121.   Cohen, S.R., and Gutstein, H.S., Spinal fluid
        differences in experimental allergic en-
        cephalomyelitis and multiple sclerosis, Science
        199, 301-303, 1978.
122.   Day, E.D., Radioimmunoassays for myelin basic
        protein, Clin. Immunol. Newsletter 3, 53-59, 1982.
123.   Bernard, C.C.A., Randell, V.B., Horvath, L.B.,
        Carnegie, P.R., and Mackay, I.R., Antibody to

myelin basic protein in extracts of multiple sclerosis brain, Immunol. 43, 447-457, 1981.

124. Wajgt, A., and Gorny, M., CSF antibodies to myelin basic protein and to myelin-associated glycoprotein in multiple sclerosis. Evidence of the intrathecal production of antibodies, Acta Neurol. Scand., 68, 337-343, 1983.

125. Bernard, C.C.A., Williamson, H.G., Randell, V.B., Lim, C.F., and Carnegie, P.R., Antibodies to viruses and myelin basic protein in multiple sclerosis and hypomyelinogenesis congenita (Hairy Shaker Disease) of lambs, in New Approaches to Nerve and Muscle Disorders. Basic and Applied Contributions, Kidman, A.D., Tomkins, J.K., and Westerman, R.A., eds, Excerpta Medica, Amsterdam-Oxford-Princeton, 1981, pp. 310-323.

126. Paterson, P.Y., Day, E.D., Whitacre, C.C., Berenberg, R.A., and Harter, D.H., Endogenous myelin basic protein-serum factors (MBP-SFs) and anti-MBP antibodies in humans. Occurrence in sera of clinically well subjects and patients with multiple sclerosis, J. Neurol. Sci. 52, 37-51, 1981.

127. Frick, E., and Stickl, H., Antibody-dependent lymphocyte cytotoxicity against basic protein of myelin in multiple sclerosis, J. Neurolog. Sciences 46, 187-197, 1980.

128. Frick, E., and Stickl, H., Specificity of antibody-dependent lymphocyte cytotoxicity against cerebral tissue constituents in multiple sclerosis. Studies with basic protein of myelin, en-cephalitogenic peptide, cerebrosides and ganglio-sides, Acta Neurol. Scand. 65, 30-37, 1982.

129. Day, E.D., Varitek, V.A., and Paterson, P.Y., Endogenous myelin basic protein-serum factors (MBP-SFs) in Lewis rats, J. Neurolog. Sciences 49, 1-17, 1981.

130. Day, E.D., Meier, H., Alpert, S.E., Varitek, V.A., Jr., and Paterson, P.Y. Comparative levels of endogenous myelin basic protein-serum factors (MBP-SFs) in adult and suckling mice (B6CBAF$_1$ and B6C3HF$_1$ strains) and in neurologically mutant mice of the same genetic background, J. Neurolog. Sciences 56, 99-105, 1982.

131. Day, E.D., Varitek, V.A., Fujinami, R.S., and Paterson, P.Y., MBP-SF, a prominent serum factor in suckling Lewis rats that additively inhibits the primary binding of myelin basic protein (MBP) to syngeneic anti-MBP antibodies, Immunochem. 15, 1-9, 1978.

132. Day, E.D., Varitek, V.A., and Paterson, P.Y.,
      Myelin basic protein serum factor (MBP-SF) in adult
      Lewis rats: a method for detection and evidence
      that MBP-SF influences the appearance of antibody
      to MBP in animals developing experimental allergic
      encephalomyelitis, Immunochem. 15, 437-442, 1978.

133. Varitek, V.A., Day, E.D., and Paterson, P.Y., Early
      loss, reappearance, and extended half-life of
      circulating antibody activity to myelin basic
      protein (MBP) in passively immunized Lewis rats:
      further evidence for accessible endogenous MBP
      neuroantigens, Mol. Immunol. 17, 127-133, 1980.

134. Rauch, H.C., and Raffel, S., Immunofluorescent
      localization of encephalitogenic protein in myelin,
      J. Immunol. 92, 452-455, 1964.

135. Sternberger, N.H., Patterns of oligodendrocyte
      function seen by immunocytochemistry, in Oligo-
      dendroglia, Norton, W.T., ed. (Adv. Neurochem.,
      vol. 5), Plenum Press, New York, 1984, pp. 125-173.

136. Sternberger, N.H., Itoyama, Y., Kies, M.W., and
      Webster, H.deF., Immunocytochemical method to
      identify basic protein in myelin-forming oligo-
      dendrocytes of newborn rat C.N.S., J. Neurocytology
      7, 251-263, 1978.

137. Sternberger, N.H., Itoyama, Y., Kies, M.W., and
      Webster, H.deF., Myelin basic protein demonstrated
      immunocytochemically in oligodendroglia prior to
      myelin sheath formation, Proc. Natl. Acad. Sci. USA
      75, 2521-2524, 1978.

138. Dupouey, P., Jacque, C., Bourne, J.M., Cesselin,
      F., Privat, A., and Baumann, N., Immunochemical
      studies of myelin basic protein in Shiverer mouse
      devoid of major dense line of myelin, Neuroscience
      Letters 12, 113-118, 1979.

139. Guarnieri, M., Himmelstein, J., and McKhann, G.M.,
      Isolated myelin quantitatively adsorbs antibody to
      basic protein, Brain Res. 72, 172-176, 1974.

140. Patterson, D.S.P., Sweasey, D., and Harkness, J.W.,
      Anti-myelin antibodies in the serum of lambs with
      experimental Border disease, J. Neurochem. 29,
      753-755, 1977.

141. Silverstein, A.M., Uhr, J.W., Kramer, K.L., and
      Lukes, R.J., Fetal response to antigenic stimulus.
      II. Antibody production by the fetal lambs. J.
      Exp. Med. 117, 799-812, 1963.

142. Halliday, R., Some factors influencing
      immunoglobulin transfer in sheep, In Maternofoetal
      Transmissions of Immunoglobulins, Hemmings, W.A.,
      ed. Cambridge University Press, 1976, pp. 409-415.

143.   McClure, S., and McCullagh, The paradox of the
        foetal lamb: immunological immaturity without
        susceptibility to tolerance induction, In Immun-
        ology of the Sheep, Borris, B., and Mujasaku, M.,
        eds., Hoffman- LaRoche & Co., Basel, Switzerland,
        1985, pp. 111-126.

144.   Potter, N.T., Hashim, G.A., and Day, E.D., Shared
        self-determinants of myelin basic protein not
        subject to evolutionary pressures. Int. J. Devel.
        Neuroscience, 6, 105-107, 1988.

145.   Kies, M.W., Species specificity and localization of
        encephalitogenic sites in myelin basic protein.
        Springer Semin. Immunopathol. 8, 295-303, 1985.

146.   Jemmerson, R., and Margoliash, E., Specificity of
        the antibody response of rabbits to a self-antigen,
        Nature 282, 468-471, 1979.

147.   Benjamin, D.C., Berzofsky, J.A., East, I.J., Gurd,
        F.R.N., Hannum, C., Leach, S.J., Margoliash, E.,
        Michael, J.G., Miller, A., Prager, E.M., Reichlin,
        M., Sercarz, E.E., Smith-Gill, S.J., Todd, P.E.,
        and Wilson, A.C., The antigenic structure of pro-
        teins: a reappraisal, Ann. Rev. Immunol. 2, 67-101,
        1984.

148.   Folch, J., and Lees, M., Proteolipids, a new type
        of tissue lipoprotein, J. Biol. Chem. 191, 807-817,
        1951.

149.   Agrawal, H.C., Hartman, B.K., Shearer, W.T.,
        Kalmbach, S., and Margolis, F.L., Purification and
        immunohistochemical localization of rat brain
        myelin proteolipid protein, J. Neurochem. 28,
        495-508, 1977.

150.   Hartman, B.K., Agrawal, H.C., Agrawal, D., and
        Kalmbach, S., Development and maturation of central
        nervous system myelin: comparison of immuno-
        histochemical localization of proteolipid protein
        and basic protein in myelin and oligodendrocytes,
        Proc. Natl. Acad. Sci. USA 79, 4217-4220, 1982.

151.   Lees, M.B., and Brostoff, S.W., Proteins of myelin,
        In Myelin, 2nd edition, Morell, P., ed., Plenum
        Press, New York, 1984, pp. 197-224.

152.   Wood, D.D., Orange, R.P., and Moscarello, M.A., The
        interaction of antibodies to two myelin proteins,
        Immunol. Communications 4, 17-27, 1975.

153.   Hampson, D.R., and Poduslo, S.E., Purification of
        proteolipid protein and production of specific
        antiserum, J. Neuroimmunol. 11, 117-129, 1986.

154.   Macklin, W.B., Braun, P.E., and Lees, M.B.,
        Electroblot analysis of the myelin proteolipid
        protein. J. Neurosci. Res. 7, 1- , 1982.

155. Trotter, J.L., Lieberman, L., Margolis, F.L., and Agrawal, H.C., Radioimmunoassay for central nervous system myelin-specific proteolipid protein, J. Neurochem. 36, 1256-1262, 1981.

156. Agrawal, H.C., and Hartman, B., Specificity of CNS myelin proteolipid and basic protein, In Biochemistry of Brain, Kamar, S., ed., Pergamon Press, New York, 1980, pp. 583-615.

157. Trifilieff, E., Luu, B., Nussbaum, J.L., Roussel, G., Espinosa de los Monteras, A., Sabatier, J.M., and Van Rietschoten, J., A specific immunological probe for the major myelin proteolipid, confirmation of a deletion in DM-20, FEBS Letters 198, 235-239, 1986.

158. Lin, L.F.H., and Lees, M.B., An immunologic probe for a defined region of the myelin proteolipid, J. Biol. Chem. 260, 4371-4377, 1985.

159. Nussbaum, J.L., Roussel, G., Wünsch, E., and Jollès, P., Site-specific antibodies to rat myelin proteolipids, directed against the C-terminal hexapeptide, J. Neurolog. Sciences 68, 89-100, 1985.

160. Laursen, R.A., Samiullah, M., and Lees, M.B., The structure of bovine brain myelin proteolipid and its organization in myelin, Proc. Natl. Acad. Sci. USA 81, 2912-2916, 1984.

161. Stoffel, W., Hillen, H., and Giersiefen, H., Structure and molecular arrangement of proteolipid protein of central nervous system myelin, Proc. Natl. Acad. Sci. USA 81, 5012-5016, 1984.

162. Nussbaum, J.L., and Roussel, G., Immunocytochemical demonstration of the transport of myelin proteolipids through the Golgi apparatus, Cell Tissue Res. 234, 547-559, 1983.

163. Van der Veen, R.C., Sobel, R.A., and Lees, M.B., Chronic experimental allergic encephalomyelitis and antibody responses in rabbits immunized with bovine proteolipid apoprotein, J. Neuroimmunol. 11, 321-333, 1986.

164. Macklin, W.B., and Lees, M.B., Solid-phase immunoassays for quantitation of antibody to bovine proteolipid apoprotein., J. Neurochem. 38, 348-355, 1982.

165. Nussbaum, J.L., Delaunoy, J.P., and Mandel, P., Some immunochemical characteristics of W1 and W2 Wolfgram protein isolated from rat brain myelin, J. Neurochem. 28, 183-191, 1977.

166. Roussel, G., Delaunoy, J.P., Nussbaum, J.L., and Mandel, P., Immunohistochemical localization of

Wolfgram proteins in nervous tissue of rat brain, Neuroscience 2, 307-313, 1977.

167.   Delaunoy, J.P., Roussel, G., Nussbaum, J.L., and Mandel, P., Immunohistochemical studies of Wolfgram proteins in central nervous system of neurological mutant mice, Brain Res. 133, 29-36, 1977.

168.   Johnson, D., Quarles, R.H., and Brady, R.O., A radioimmunoassay for the myelin-associated glyco-proteins, J. Neurochem. 39, 1356-1361, 1982.

169.   Quarles, R.H., Johnson, D., Brady, R.O., and Sternberger, N.H., Preparation and characterization of antisera to the myelin-associated glycoprotein, Neurochem. Res. 6, 1115-1127, 1981.

170.   Poduslo, J.F., and McFarlin, D.E., Immunogenicity of a membrane surface glycoprotein associated with central nervous system myelin, Brain Res. 159, 234-238, 1978.

171.   Sternberger, N.H., Quarles, R.H., Itoyama, Y., and Webster, H.deF., Myelin-associated glycoprotein demonstrated immunocytochemically in myelin and myelin-forming cells of developing rat, Proc. Natl. Acad. Sci. USA 76, 1510-1514, 1979.

172.   Itoyama, Y., Sternberger, N.H., Webster, D.deF., Quarles, R.H., Cohen, S.R., and Richardson, E.P., Jr., Immunocytochemical observations on the dis-tribution of myelin-associated glycoprotein and myelin basic protein in multiple sclerosis lesions, Ann. Neurol. 7, 167-177, 1980.

173.   Sternberger, N.H., McFarlin, D.E., Traugott, U., and Raine, C.S., Myelin basic protein and myelin-associated glycoprotein in chronic, relapsing experimental allergic encephalomyelitis, J. Neuro-immunol. 6, 217-229, 1984.

174.   Trapp, B.D., and Quarles, R.H., Immunocytochemical localization of the myelin-associated glycoprotein. Fact or artifact? J. Neuroimmunol. 6, 231-249, 1984.

175.   Prineas, J.W., Kwon, E.D., Sternberger, N.H., and Lennon, V.A., The distribution of myelin-associated glycoprotein and myelin basic protein in actively demyelinating multiple sclerosis lesions, J. Neuro-immunol. 6, 251-264, 1984.

176.   Steck, A.J., Murray, N., Vandevelde, M., and Zurbriggen, A., Human monoclonal antibodies to myelin-associated glycoprotein. Comparison of specificity and use for immunocytochemical locali-zation of the antigen, J. Neuroimmunol. 5, 145-156, 1983.

177.   O'Shannessy, D.J., Willison, H.J., Inuzuka, T., Debersen, M.J., and Quarles, R.H., The species

distribution of nervous system antigens that react with anti-myelin-associated glycoprotein antibodies, J. Neuroimmunol. 9, 255-268, 1985.

178. Wajgt, A., Gorny, M.K,., and Jenek, R., The influence of high dose prednisone medication on autoantibody specific activity and on circulating immune complex levels in cerebrospinal fluid of patients with multiple sclerosis, Acta Neurolog. Scand. 68, 378-385, 1983.

179. Nobile-Orazio, E., Spagnol, G., and Scarlato, G., Failure to detect anti-MAG antibodies by RIA in CSF of patients with multiple sclerosis, J. Neuroimmunol. 11, 165-169, 1986.

180. Dal Canto, M.C., and Barbano, R.L., Antibody to myelin-associated glycoprotein reacts with plasma cells in mice, J. Neuroimmunol. 10, 279-286, 1986.

181. Latoo, N., Braun, P.E., Gross, R.B., Sherman, W.H., Penn, A.S., and Chess, L., Plasma cell dyscrasia and peripheral neuropathy: identification of the myelin antigens that react with human paraproteins, Proc. Natl. Acad. Sci. USA 78, 7139-7142, 1981.

182. Braun, P.E., Frail, D.E., and Latov, N., Myelin-associated glycoprotein is the antigen for a monoclonal IgM in polyneuropathy, J. Neurochem. 39, 1261-1265, 1982.

183. Favilla, J.T., Frail, D.E., Palkovits, C.G., Stoner, G.L., Braun, P.E., and Webster, H. deF., Myelin-associated glycoprotein (MAG) distribution in human central nervous system tissue studied immunocytochemically with monoclonal antibody, J. Neuroimmunol. 6, 19-30, 1984.

184. Webster, H.deF., Palkovits, C.G., Stoner, G.L., Favilla, J.T., Frail, D.E., and Braun, P.E., Myelin-associated glycoprotein--electron microscopic immunocytochemical localization in compact developing and CNS myelin, J. Neurochem. 41, 1469-1479, 1983.

185. Ilyas, A.A., Quarles, R.H., MacIntosh, T.D., Dobersen, M.J., Trapp, B.D., Dalakas, M.C., and Brady, R.O., IgM in a human neuropathy related to paraproteinemia binds to a carbohydrate determinant in the myelin- associated protein and to a ganglioside, Proc. Natl. Acad. Sci. USA 81, 1225-1229, 1984.

186. Nobile-Orazio, E., Hays, A.P., Latov, N., Perman, G., Golier, J., Shy, M.E., and Freddo, L., Specificity of mouse and human monoclonal antibodies to myelin-associated glycoprotein, Neurology 34, 1336-1342, 1984.

187. Murray, N., Steck, A.J., Page, N., and Perruisseau, G., Human monoclonal antibodies to myelin-associated glycoprotein are directed against the polypeptide and not the carbohydrate moiety, J. Neuroimmunol. 7, 21-26, 1984/85.

188. Frail, D.E., Edwards, A.M., and Braun, P.E., Molecular characteristics of the epitope in myelin-associated glycoprotein that is recognized by a monoclonal IgM in human neuropathy patients, Mol. Immunol. 21, 721-725, 1984.

189. Linnington, C., Webb, M., and Woodhams, P.L., A novel myelin-associated glycoprotein defined by a mouse monoclonal antibody, J. Neuroimmunol. 6, 387-396, 1984.

190. Dumas, M., Zurbriggen, A., Vandevelde, M., Yim, S.H., Arnason, B.G.W., Szuchet, S., and Meier, C., J. Neuroimmunol. 9, 55-67, 1985.

191. Rapport, M.M., Lipid Haptens, In Handbook of Neurochemistry, Vol. 3, Lijtha, A. (ed.), Plenum Press, New York, 1970, pp. 509-524.

192. Brandt, R., Guth, H., and Müller, R., ZurFrage der Organspezifität von Lipoidintikörpern, Klin. Wochschr. 5, 655, 1926.

193. Witebsky, E., and Steinfeld, J., Untersuchungan über spezifische Antigenfunctionen von Organen, Z. Immunitätsforsch. 58, 271-296, 1928.

194. Joffe, S., Rapport, M.M., and Graf., L., Immunochemical studies of organ and tumor lipids XII. Identification of an organ specific lipid hapten in brain, Nature 197, 60-62, 1963.

195. Rapport, M.M., Graf, L., Autilio, L.A., and Norton, W.T., Immunochemical studies of organ and tumor lipids XIV. Galactocerebroside determinants in the myelin sheath of the central nervous system, J. Neurochem. 11, 855-864, 1964.

196. Gregson, N.A., Kennedy, M., and Leibowitz, S., The specificity of anti-galactocerebroside antibody and its reaction with lysolecithin-solubilized myelin, Immunol. 26, 743-757, 1974.

197. Oxberry, J.M., and Gregson, N.A., The agglutination of myelin suspension by specific antisera, Brain Res. 78, 303-313, 1974.

198. Fry, J.M., Lisak, R.P., Manning, M.C., and Silberberg, D.H., Serological techniques for detection of antibody to galactocerebroside, J. Immunol. Meth. 11, 195-193, 1976.

199. Tabira, T., and Endoh, M., Humoral immune responses to myelin basic protein, cerebroside and ganglioside in chronic relapsing experimental allergic

encephalomyelitis of the guinea pig, J. Neurol. Sci. 67, 201-212, 1985.

200. Hakomori, S.I., Preparation and properties of anti-sulfatide serum, J. Immunol. 112, 424-426, 1974.

201. Zalc, B., Jacque, C., Radin, N.S., and Dupouey, P., Immunogenicity of sulfatide, Immunochem. 14, 775-779, 1977.

202. Dupouey, P., Zalc, B., Lefroit-Joly, M., and Gomes, D., Localization of galactosylceramide and sulfatide at the surface of the myelin sheath: An immunofluorescence study in liquid medium, Cell. Mol. Biol. 25, 269-272, 1979.

203. Uemara, K.I., Yazawa-Watanebe, M., Kitazawa, N., and Taketomi, T., Immunochemical studies of lipids VI. Reactions of anti-sulfatide antibodies with sulfatide in liposomal and myelin membranes, J. Biochem. 87, 1221-1227, 1980.

204. Ledeen, R.W., and Yu, R.K., Ganglioside structure, isolation, and analysis, Meth. Enzymol. 83, 139-191, 1982.

205. Jacobson, R.I., Kasai, N., Richards, F.F., and Yu, R.K., Preparation of anti-G_{M4} antiserum and its assay by a solid-phase radioimmunoassay J. Neuroimmunol. 3, 225-235, 1982.

206. Norton, W.T., and Cammer, W., Isolation and characterization of myelin, In Myelin, 2nd Edition, Morell, P. (ed.), Plenum Press, New York, 1984, pp. 147-195.

207. Saito, M., and Rosenberg, A., Sialosylgalactosylceramide (G_{M4}) is a major ganglioside in chicken embryonic liver, J. Lipid Res. 23, 9-19, 1982.

208. Cochran, F.B., Jr., Yu, R.K., and Ledeen, R.W., Myelin gangliosides in vertebrates, J. Neurochem. 39, 773-779, 1982.

209. Naiki, M., Marcus, D.M., and Ledeen, R., Properties of antisera to ganglioside G_{M1} and asialo G_{M1}, J. Immunol. 113, 84-93, 1974.

210. Gregson, N.A., and Hammer, C.T., Some immunological properties of antisera raised against the trisialoganglioside GT_{1b}, Mol. Immunol. 19, 543-550, 1982.

211. Kusonoki, S., Tsuzi, S., and Nagai, Y., Ganglio-N-tetraosylceramide (asialo GM_1), an antigen common to the brain and immune system: its localization in myelin, Brain Res. 334, 117-124, 1985.

212. Kasai, M., Iwamori, M., Nagai, Y., Okimura, K., and Tada, T., A glycolipid on the surface of natural killer cells, Europ. J. Immunol. 10, 175-180, 1980.

213. Golub, E.S., and Day, E.D., Localization of brain-associated hematopoietic antigens in the neuronal

fraction of brain, Cell. Immunol. 15, 427-431, 1975.

214.   Gregson, N.A., and Oxberry, J.M., An immunochemical investigation of ganglioside in rat brain myelin, Biochem. Soc. Trans. 4, 310-311, 1976.

215.   Arnon, R., Crisp, E., Kelley, R., Ellison, G.W., Myers, L.W., and Tourtelotte, W.W., Anti-ganglioside antibodies in multiple sclerosis, J. Neurol. Sci. 46, 179-186, 1980.

216.   Bornstein, M.B., and Appel, S.H., The application of tissue culture to the study of experimental 'allergic' encephalomyelitis. I. Patterns of demyelination, J. Neuropathol. Exp. Neurol. 20, 141-157, 1961.

217.   Appel, S.H., and Bornstein, M.B., The application of tissue cultures to the study of experimental allergic encephalomyelitis. II. Serum factors responsible for deymyelination, J. Exp. Med. 119, 303-312, 1964.

218.   Bornstein, M.B., and Raine, C.S., Experimental allergic encephalomyelitis. Antiserum inhibition of myelination in vitro, Lab. Invest. 23, 536-542, 1970.

219.   Dorfman, S.H., Holtzer, H., and Silberberg, D.H., Effect of 5-bromo-2'- deoxyuridine or cytosine-B-D-arabinofuranoside hydrochloride on myelination in newborn rat cerebellum cultures following removal of myelination inhibiting antiserum to whole cord or cerebroside, Brain Res. 104, 283-293, 1976.

220.   Dubois-Dalcq, M., Niedick, B., and Buyse, M., Action of anti-cerebroside on myelinated nervous tissue culture. Pathol. Europ. 5, 331-347, 1970.

221.   Fry, J.M., Weissbarth, S., Lehrer, G.M., and Bornstein, M.B., Cerebroside antibody inhibits sulfatide synthesis and myelination and demyelination in cord tissue cultures, Science 183, 540-542, 1974.

222.   Hruby, S., Alvord, E.C., Jr., and Seil, F.J., Synthetic galacto- cerebrosides evoke myelination-inhibiting antibodies, Science 14, 173-175, 1977.

223.   Dorfman, S.H., Fry, J.M., Silberberg, D.H., Crose, C., and Manning, M.C., Cerebroside antibody titers in antisera capable of myelination inhibition and demyelination, Brain Res. 147, 410-415, 1978.

224.   Raine, C.S., Johnson, A.B., Marcus, D.M., Suzuki, A., and Bornstein, M.B., Demyelination in vitro. Absorption studies demonstrate that galac-

tocerebroside is a major target, J. Neurolog. Sci. 52, 117-131, 1981.

225. Seil, F.J., and Agrawal, H.C., Myelin-proteolipid protein does not induce demyelinating or myelination-inhibiting antibodies, Brain Res. 194, 273-277, 1980.

226. Seil, F.J., Quarles, R.H., Johnson, D., and Brady, R.O., Immunization with purified myelin-associated glycoprotein does not evoke myelination inhibiting or demyelinating antibodies, Brain Res. 209, 470-475, 1981.

227. Johnson, A.B., and Bornstein, B.M., Myelin-binding antibodies in vitro Immunoperoxidase studies with experimental allergic encephalomyelitis, anti-galactocerebroside, and multiple sclerosis sera, Brain Res. 159, 173-182, 1978.

228. Grundkl-Iqbal, I., and Bornstein, M.B., Multiple sclerosis: immunochemical studies on the demyelinating serum factor, Brain Res., 160, 489-503, 1979.

229. Lebar, R., Boutry, J.M., Vincent, C., Robineaux, R., and Voisin, G.A., Studies on autoimmune encephalomyelitis in the guinea pig II. An in vitro investigation on the nature, properties, and specificity of the serum-demyelinating factor, J. Immunol. 116, 1439-1446, 1976.

230. Abramsky, O., Lisak, R.P., Silberberg, D.H., Pleasure, D.E., and George, J., Antibodies to oligodendroglia in patients with multiple sclerosis, N. Eng. J. Med. 297, 1207-1211, 1977.

231. Abramsky, O., Lisak, R.P., Pleasure, D., Gilden, D.H., and Silberberg, D.H., Immunologic characterization of oligodendroglia, Neurosci. Letters 8, 311-316, 1978.

232. Appel, H., Antibodies to oligodendroglia in multiple sclerosis, N. Eng. J. Med. 298, 743 (Letter), 1978.

233. Abramsky, O., Saida, T., Lisak, R.P., Pleasure, D., and Silberberg, D.H., Immunologic studies with isolated oligodendrocytes, Neurol. 27, 342-343, 1977.

234. Traugott, U., Snyder, D.S., Norton, W.E., and Raine, C.S., Characterization of anti-oligodendrocyte serum, Ann. Neurol. 4, 431-439, 1978.

235. Rostami, A., Pleasure, D.E., Lisak, R.P., Silberberg, D.H., Abramsky, O., and Phillips, S.M., Radioimmunoassay for detection of anti- oligodendrocyte antibodies, Neurosci. Letters 23, 143-148, 1981.

236.   Roussel, G., and Nussbaum, J.L., Immunohisto-
         chemical study with an anti-myelin serum, a marker
         for all glial cells except 'dark' oligodendrocytes,
         J. Neuroimmunol. 5, 209-226, 1983.
237.   Lebar, R., and Lees, M.B., Dot immunobinding as a
         tool for the study of the CNS myelin antigen, M_2, J.
         Neuroimmunol. 8, 43-55, 1985.
238.   Gregson, N.A., Kennedy, M.C., and Leibowitz, S.,
         Immunological reactions with lysolecithin-solubil-
         ized myelin, Immunol. 20, 501-512, 1971.
239.   Day, E.D., Myelin as a locus for radioantibody
         absorption in vivo in brain and brain tumors,
         Cancer Res. 28, 1335-1343, 1968.
240.   Day, E.D., and Appel, S.H., The biologic half-life
         of brain-localized anti-synapse radioantibodies, J.
         Immunol. 104, 710-717, 1970.
241.   Day, E.D., Rigsbee, L., Wilkins, R., and Mahaley,
         M.S., Jr., Localization of anti-brain radio-
         antibodies in rat brain, J. Immunol. 98, 62-66,
         1967.
242.   Day, E.D., and Rigsbee, L.C., Distribution analysis
         of brain-localized radioantibodies after zonal
         ultracentrifugation in a sucrose density- gradient,
         J. Immunol. 103, 556-558, 1969.
243.   McMillan, P.N., Mickey, D.D., Kaufman, B., and Day,
         E.D., The specificity and cross-reactivity of
         antimyelin antibodies as determined by sequential
         adsorption analysis. J. Immunol. 107, 1611-1617,
         1971.

Index